T0312870

Modeling to Inform Infectious Disease Control

Chapman & Hall/CRC Biostatistics Series

Published Titles

Adaptive Design Methods in Clinical Trials, Second Edition
Shein-Chung Chow and Mark Chang

Adaptive Designs for Sequential Treatment Allocation
Alessandro Baldi Antognini and Alessandra Giovagnoli

Adaptive Design Theory and Implementation Using SAS and R, Second Edition
Mark Chang

Advanced Bayesian Methods for Medical Test Accuracy
Lyle D. Broemeling

Advances in Clinical Trial Biostatistics
Nancy L. Geller

Applied Meta-Analysis with R
Ding-Geng (Din) Chen and Karl E. Peace

Basic Statistics and Pharmaceutical Statistical Applications, Second Edition
James E. De Muth

Bayesian Adaptive Methods for Clinical Trials
Scott M. Berry, Bradley P. Carlin, J. Jack Lee, and Peter Muller

Bayesian Analysis Made Simple: An Excel GUI for WinBUGS
Phil Woodward

Bayesian Methods for Measures of Agreement
Lyle D. Broemeling

Bayesian Methods in Epidemiology
Lyle D. Broemeling

Bayesian Methods in Health Economics
Gianluca Baio

Bayesian Missing Data Problems: EM, Data Augmentation and Noniterative Computation
Ming T. Tan, Guo-Liang Tian, and Kai Wang Ng

Bayesian Modeling in Bioinformatics
Dipak K. Dey, Samiran Ghosh, and Bani K. Mallick

Benefit-Risk Assessment in Pharmaceutical Research and Development
Andreas Sashegyi, James Felli, and Rebecca Noel

Biosimilars: Design and Analysis of Follow-on Biologics
Shein-Chung Chow

Biostatistics: A Computing Approach
Stewart J. Anderson

Causal Analysis in Biomedicine and Epidemiology: Based on Minimal Sufficient Causation
Mikel Aickin

Clinical and Statistical Considerations in Personalized Medicine
Claudio Carini, Sandeep Menon, and Mark Chang

Clinical Trial Data Analysis using R
Ding-Geng (Din) Chen and Karl E. Peace

Clinical Trial Methodology
Karl E. Peace and Ding-Geng (Din) Chen

Computational Methods in Biomedical Research
Ravindra Khattree and Dayanand N. Naik

Computational Pharmacokinetics
Anders Källén

Confidence Intervals for Proportions and Related Measures of Effect Size
Robert G. Newcombe

Controversial Statistical Issues in Clinical Trials
Shein-Chung Chow

Data and Safety Monitoring Committees in Clinical Trials
Jay Herson

Design and Analysis of Animal Studies in Pharmaceutical Development
Shein-Chung Chow and Jen-pei Liu

Design and Analysis of Bioavailability and Bioequivalence Studies, Third Edition
Shein-Chung Chow and Jen-pei Liu

Design and Analysis of Bridging Studies
Jen-pei Liu, Shein-Chung Chow, and Chin-Fu Hsiao

Design and Analysis of Clinical Trials for Predictive Medicine
Shigeyuki Matsui, Marc Buyse, and Richard Simon

Design and Analysis of Clinical Trials with Time-to-Event Endpoints
Karl E. Peace

Design and Analysis of Non-Inferiority Trials
Mark D. Rothmann, Brian L. Wiens, and Ivan S. F. Chan

Difference Equations with Public Health Applications
Lemuel A. Moyé and Asha Seth Kapadia

DNA Methylation Microarrays: Experimental Design and Statistical Analysis
Sun-Chong Wang and Arturas Petronis

DNA Microarrays and Related Genomics Techniques: Design, Analysis, and Interpretation of Experiments
David B. Allison, Grier P. Page, T. Mark Beasley, and Jode W. Edwards

Dose Finding by the Continual Reassessment Method
Ying Kuen Cheung

Elementary Bayesian Biostatistics
Lemuel A. Moyé

Frailty Models in Survival Analysis
Andreas Wienke

Generalized Linear Models: A Bayesian Perspective
Dipak K. Dey, Sujit K. Ghosh, and Bani K. Mallick

Handbook of Regression and Modeling: Applications for the Clinical and Pharmaceutical Industries
Daryl S. Paulson

Inference Principles for Biostatisticians
Ian C. Marschner

Interval-Censored Time-to-Event Data: Methods and Applications
Ding-Geng (Din) Chen, Jianguo Sun, and Karl E. Peace

Joint Models for Longitudinal and Time-to-Event Data: With Applications in R
Dimitris Rizopoulos

Measures of Interobserver Agreement and Reliability, Second Edition
Mohamed M. Shoukri

Medical Biostatistics, Third Edition
A. Indrayan

Meta-Analysis in Medicine and Health Policy
Dalene Stangl and Donald A. Berry

Mixed Effects Models for the Population Approach: Models, Tasks, Methods and Tools
Marc Lavielle

Modeling to Inform Infectious Disease Control
Niels G. Becker

Monte Carlo Simulation for the Pharmaceutical Industry: Concepts, Algorithms, and Case Studies
Mark Chang

Multiple Testing Problems in Pharmaceutical Statistics
Alex Dmitrienko, Ajit C. Tamhane, and Frank Bretz

Noninferiority Testing in Clinical Trials: Issues and Challenges
Tie-Hua Ng

Optimal Design for Nonlinear Response Models
Valerii V. Fedorov and Sergei L. Leonov

Patient-Reported Outcomes: Measurement, Implementation and Interpretation
Joseph C. Cappelleri, Kelly H. Zou, Andrew G. Bushmakin, Jose Ma. J. Alvir, Demissie Alemayehu, and Tara Symonds

Quantitative Evaluation of Safety in Drug Development: Design, Analysis and Reporting
Qi Jiang and H. Amy Xia

Randomized Clinical Trials of Nonpharmacological Treatments
Isabelle Boutron, Philippe Ravaud, and David Moher

Randomized Phase II Cancer Clinical Trials
Sin-Ho Jung

Sample Size Calculations for Clustered and Longitudinal Outcomes in Clinical Research
Chul Ahn, Moonseong Heo, and Song Zhang

Sample Size Calculations in Clinical Research, Second Edition
Shein-Chung Chow, Jun Shao and Hansheng Wang

Statistical Analysis of Human Growth and Development
Yin Bun Cheung

Statistical Design and Analysis of Stability Studies
Shein-Chung Chow

Statistical Evaluation of Diagnostic Performance: Topics in ROC Analysis
Kelly H. Zou, Aiyi Liu, Andriy Bandos, Lucila Ohno-Machado, and Howard Rockette

Statistical Methods for Clinical Trials
Mark X. Norleans

Statistical Methods in Drug Combination Studies
Wei Zhao and Harry Yang

Statistics in Drug Research: Methodologies and Recent Developments
Shein-Chung Chow and Jun Shao

Statistics in the Pharmaceutical Industry, Third Edition
Ralph Buncher and Jia-Yeong Tsay

Survival Analysis in Medicine and Genetics
Jialiang Li and Shuangge Ma

Theory of Drug Development
Eric B. Holmgren

Translational Medicine: Strategies and Statistical Methods
Dennis Cosmatos and Shein-Chung Chow

Chapman & Hall/CRC Biostatistics Series

Modeling to Inform Infectious Disease Control

Niels G. Becker
Australian National University
Canberra, Australia

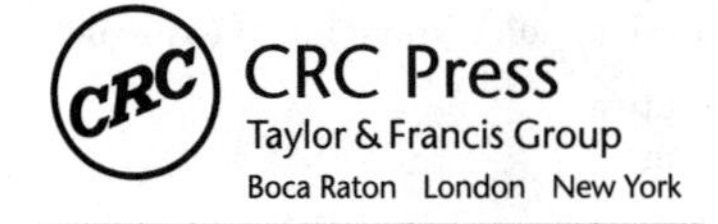

CRC Press is an imprint of the
Taylor & Francis Group, an **informa** business
A CHAPMAN & HALL BOOK

CRC Press
Taylor & Francis Group
6000 Broken Sound Parkway NW, Suite 300
Boca Raton, FL 33487-2742

Printed on acid-free paper
Version Date: 20150227

International Standard Book Number-13: 978-1-4987-3106-5 (Hardback)

Visit the Taylor & Francis Web site at
http://www.taylorandfrancis.com

and the CRC Press Web site at
http://www.crcpress.com

Contents

Preface **xi**

1 Introduction **1**
1.1 Motivation 1
1.2 Terminology 1
1.3 Scope and layout of the book 4
1.4 Bibliographic notes 6

2 Minor outbreaks when infectives are homogeneous **7**
2.1 When are outbreaks certain to be minor? 7
2.2 Preventing epidemics by mass immunization 8
2.3 Reproduction number 9
2.4 What is a minor outbreak? 13
2.5 Probability of a minor outbreak 16
2.6 Importation of the infectious disease 19
2.7 Estimating R 20
2.8 Discussion 23
2.9 Exercises 27
2.10 Supplementary material 30
2.11 Bibliographic notes 36

3 Minor outbreaks in a community of households **37**
3.1 Modified allocation of offspring 37
3.2 Household reproduction number 38
3.3 When are outbreaks certain to be minor? 40
3.4 Mass immunization 40
3.5 Are results affected by the way the infection is imported? 44
3.6 Estimating R_{H} 46
3.7 Discussion 46
3.8 Exercises 48
3.9 Supplementary material 50
3.10 Bibliographic notes 54

4 Minor outbreaks when individuals differ **55**
4.1 Type-specific offspring distributions 55
4.2 When are outbreaks certain to be minor? 56
4.3 Mass immunization 57
4.4 Types of individual in a community of households 60
4.5 Two reproduction numbers for a community of households 61
4.6 Discussion 63
4.7 Exercises 65
4.8 Supplementary material 68
4.9 Bibliographic notes 70

5 Transmission intensity function **71**
5.1 Describing transmission intensity by a function 71
5.2 Estimating the transmission intensity function 73
5.3 Role of the transmission intensity function in modeling 75
5.4 Discussion 79
5.5 Exercises 80
5.6 Supplementary material 85
5.7 Bibliographic notes 89

6 Partially effective vaccines **91**
6.1 Vaccine effect on transmission between individuals 91
6.2 Impact of mass immunization on the reproduction number 94
6.3 Estimating vaccine effects 96
6.4 Discussion 97
6.5 Exercises 99
6.6 Supplementary material 101
6.7 Bibliographic notes 102

7 Social distancing **103**
7.1 What is social distancing? 103
7.2 Reduced mixing 104
7.3 Isolating symptomatic infectives 106
7.4 Targeting high transmission intensities 109
7.5 Discussion 115
7.6 Exercises 116
7.7 Supplementary material 118
7.8 Bibliographic notes 119

8 Reducing epidemic size **121**
8.1 Simulated epidemics 121
8.2 The nature of our deterministic epidemic model 123
8.3 Epidemic size in a homogeneous community 123
8.4 Mass immunization 125

8.5 Herd immunity 128
8.6 Estimating the reproduction number 130
8.7 Types of individual 132
8.8 Discussion 139
8.9 Exercises 140
8.10 Supplementary material 144
8.11 Bibliographic notes 150

9 Dynamics of infection incidence 151
9.1 The epidemic curve 151
9.2 Estimating parameter values from daily incidence data 154
9.3 Endemic transmission 160
9.4 Discussion 162
9.5 Exercises 164
9.6 Supplementary material 166
9.7 Bibliographic notes 168

10 Using data to inform model choice 169
10.1 Model-free comparison of data on outbreak size 169
10.2 Transmission among homogeneous individuals 172
10.3 Allowing transmission rates to differ between individuals 175
10.4 Discussion 180
10.5 Exercises 181
10.6 Supplementary material 188
10.7 Bibliographic notes 195

Terminology and notation 197

References 201

Subject index 205

Preface

Modeling is increasingly used to inform infectious disease control. Unfortunately, the technical nature of modeling prevents public health officers from taking full advantage of models when developing strategies to mitigate infectious disease transmission. The aim of this book is

(i) to make modeling insights about the control of infectious diseases accessible to a wide audience, and
(ii) to promote an interest in modeling that is simple and clearly targeted at providing useful insights about infectious disease management.

To this end the core material of every chapter is presented in a way that requires only a modest knowledge of mathematics. For this core material, it is assumed that the reader is able to interpret an algebraic formula and understands what it means to solve an equation. Such readers will be able to use the core material to assess intervention options for the control of infectious diseases. Technical support material is deferred to a separate section at the end of each chapter, under the heading "Supplementary material," for readers with a stronger background in mathematics and an interest in learning the art of modeling towards a clear purpose.

The core material is suitable for a Master of Public Health course. A one semester course in biostatistics is a useful prerequisite for this material. Students are assisted by instructive exercises, a glossary of infectious disease terminology and a glossary of notation.

The technical material at the back of each chapter is generally partitioned into subsections. This gives instructors scope to tailor a course to the mathematical background of their students.

The author is grateful to Prof. Klaus Dietz for making the data on the outbreak of measles in Hagelloch available. I am also grateful for discussions and collaborations I have enjoyed with many colleagues. You have taught me so much.

Niels G. Becker
The Australian National University

CHAPTER 1

Introduction

1.1 Motivation

Despite much progress in the development and implementation of interventions to mitigate illness from infectious diseases, there remains a need for public health management of epidemics. This is evident from current childhood vaccination schedules, which are extensive, continue to grow and struggle to maintain adequate vaccination coverage for all the diseases they target. It is also evident from the need to respond to outbreaks following introductions of infections from outside the community, which occur all too frequently in a world where borders are increasingly porous. Further, our experiences with the human immunodeficiency virus (HIV), severe acute respiratory syndrome (SARS), the ever-present threat of pandemic influenza and outbreaks of ebola virus disease (EVD) remind us of the continuing need to be vigilant against emergence of new infectious diseases.

Ideally, strategies for the public health management of infectious diseases are guided by evidence acquired from intervention studies conducted in real communities. Unfortunately, such studies are very time consuming, resource intensive and often hampered by ethical obstacles.

Mathematical modeling is increasingly seen as a useful alternative for guiding management of infectious disease control, because it provides a way to assess an intervention relatively quickly, cheaply and safely. For example, several nations developed preparedness plans for pandemic influenza at the start of this century in close collaboration with infectious disease modelers.

This book describes a way of modeling and presents modeling results that help to guide effective management of infectious disease transmission and outbreak response. The core part of each chapter assumes that the reader is able to interpret an algebraic formula, understands what it means to solve an equation and has some familiarity with basic statistics. Technical support material is presented in a "Supplementary material" section at the back of each chapter.

As the book is intended to meet the needs of people with different backgrounds, it is useful to begin with some basic terminology.

1.2 Terminology

Throughout the book "he" should be read as "he or she."

Infectious disease and modeling terms are defined as they arise in the text and terminology is conveniently summarized in a glossary on page 197. Nevertheless, it is useful to introduce a few fundamental concepts before we begin our discussion.

Concepts of infectious disease epidemiology

By an infectious disease we mean a disease which is infectious in the sense that an infected host passes through a stage, called the *infectious period*, during which he (or she) is able to transmit the pathogen to another susceptible host, either by a direct "sufficiently close" host-to-host contact or by dispersing the pathogen in the local environment and the susceptible host then making "sufficiently close" contact with the contaminated environment. In this context the meaning of environment depends on the particular disease. The infected environment might include, for example, the linen and cutlery of a household as well as the ambient air in a commuter train.

For convenience, individuals who are susceptible to the infection are referred to as *susceptibles*. Similarly, infected individuals will be referred to as *infectives*. Mostly infective refers to an infected person who is infectious. To simplify wording, we occasionally stretch the definition of infective to include infected individuals from the time of acquiring the infection until the time when they are no longer able to transmit the pathogen.

An *infectious contact* is a contact, made by an infectious person with another individual, that is close enough to transmit the infection if the second individual is a susceptible. An infectious contact does not lead to transmission of the infection if the contacted person is immune, perhaps as result of a previous infection or vaccination.

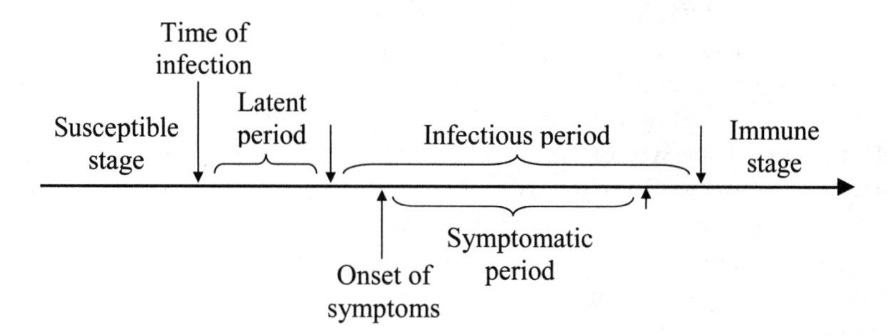

Figure 1.1 *Illustrative timeline of the stages of infection in a host.*

Figure 1.1 depicts a typical timeline for the stages through which a host passes following infection. Following the infectious contact that led to his infection, the infected host first passes through a *latent period*. During this period the infectious agent establishes itself within the host and the host is not able to transmit the infection. The infectious period is next and we assume that the infected host then becomes immune from further infection for the remaining duration of the outbreak.

Much of the material of this book looks at outbreaks arising when an infectious disease is newly introduced. For infections that have circulated previously this implies that the outbreak was preceded by a period of *elimination*. An infectious disease is said to be eliminated from a community when the community has enjoyed a case-free period long enough to preclude the presence of undetected cases in the community. The period of elimination is usually temporary, since re-introduction of the infectious disease is likely given modern rates of travel and the difficulty of preventing infected individuals from entering the community.

Elements of a model

Models describe the dynamics and eventual outcomes of disease transmission by equations expressed in terms of quantities called *parameters* and *variables*.

Each parameter is a constant. Its value is determined by characteristics of the infectious disease, characteristics of the community, or both. For example, the mean duration of the infectious period is a parameter, as is the mean rate at which pairs of individuals make contact close enough for the infection to be transmitted from one to the other. The preferred method for assigning values to parameters is to estimate them from data, perhaps using data collected in a field study or using data recorded in an infectious disease register. Estimates for parameter values should, when possible, be accompanied by a measure of the precision of the estimate. That is, a standard error or confidence interval should be provided.

Variables are quantities such as the number of community members still susceptible and the current number of infected individuals circulating. It is the behavior of the variables over time that captures the dynamics of the spread of the infectious disease.

Parameters and variables are bound together by model equations formulated to capture the mechanism that generates transmission of the infectious disease.

A model can describe the dynamics of the spread of an infectious disease fully only when all parameter values and the initial values of the variables are specified. Specifically, the variable values we need to know when an infection is freshly introduced into the community include (i) the number of infected individuals who introduced the infection, and (ii) the proportion of community members who are susceptible at start of the outbreak.

Chapter 5, and later chapters, includes models that describe the dynamics of transmission over time and introduces time-dependent public health interventions. Various concepts of *transmission intensity* arise in these models, which we define as they arise. However, to avoid confusion later, it is useful to prepare ourselves by distinguishing the different types of transmission intensity that we will encounter and to introduce the terminology for them.

The building block for these concepts is the transmission intensity between a given infective, A say, and a given susceptible, B say. The transmission intensity between this infective-susceptible pair describes how the risk of infective A transmitting the infection to susceptible B changes over time. In different discussions we refer to this as "the transmission intensity that A exerts on B" or "the transmission intensity that B is exposed to from A."

From a community perspective transmission of an infectious disease is progressed by an interaction between a group of infectives and a group of susceptibles. Specifically, at any given time, infective A exerts a transmission intensity on every susceptible in the community. Summing over these gives the *aggregated transmission intensity* A *exerts* on community susceptibles at that time. This concept is useful, for example, when describing the mean number of individuals A infects. Similarly, at any given time, susceptible B is exposed to a transmission intensity from each current community infective. Summing over these gives the *aggregated transmission intensity to which* B *is exposed* at that time. This concept is useful, for example, when describing the probability that B is infected.

Each of these transmission intensities changes over time and we will need to accumulate them over time, which leads to what we call *cumulative transmission intensity functions.* To be clear, we use the adjective "aggregated" when transmission intensities are summed over the current infectives, or the current susceptibles, at a given time, but use the adjective "cumulative" when we "sum" a specified transmission intensity over time. More precise definitions are given as we need them.

Each model is formulated to suit a specific community setting. The setting is generally specified in each discussion or exercise. The baseline community setting is a community made up of a large number of individuals who are homogeneous and mix uniformly. This setting should be assumed when a specification of the community setting has been omitted.

We sometimes specify that the size of the community is $n + 1$. The inclusion of $+1$ is merely a minor notational convenience when an outbreak starts with 1 infective and n susceptibles.

A glossary of notation is included to assist readers with the notation used for parameters and variables; see page 200.

1.3 Scope and layout of the book

The core of the chapters tells the story of the way models inform infectious disease control, avoiding technical detail as much as possible. Near the end of each chapter is a section titled *Supplementary material.* It gives supporting material of a technical nature for the benefit of readers with a stronger mathematical background, but occasionally contains additional results. This form of presentation is used in the hope that the material thereby becomes accessible to a wide audience, including epidemiologists, public health officers and individuals wanting to learn the art of purpose-focused modeling.

The topic of infectious disease modeling has grown enormously, making it necessary to restrict the material in a book of this kind. Here the focus is on the control of infectious diseases that are spread primarily by person-to-person contact. We also assume that an individual can be infected only once over the period for which the model is proposed.

New material is introduced in the simplest community setting first and is sometimes extended to allow for different types of individual and a community comprised of households. The simplest setting is generally a large community of homogeneous individuals who mix uniformly, by which we mean that

(i) every susceptible individual is equally susceptible to infection,
(ii) every infected individual has the same infectivity, and
(iii) each pair of individuals is equally likely to share a contact during any time increment.

This simplified setting is well suited for introducing concepts that are key to infectious disease control. It provides a solid base from which one can conveniently progress to more realistic community settings.

Chapters 2, 3 and 4 present material that helps us to understand the requirements for preventing epidemics. There are two reasons why this topic is a natural place to start. Firstly, preventing epidemics is the preferred outcome of public health efforts to control an infectious disease, so our material moves quickly to a major control issue. Secondly, while the focus is on preventing epidemics there is no need to incorporate "depletion in the number of susceptible community members" into the model specification. This allows us to make good progress, because we can utilize models for which a rich body of results is available.

We start in Chapter 2 with the simple setting in which all infected individuals have the same potential to infect others. The two chapters that follow add a household structure to the community and allow groups of individuals, such as children and adults, to play different roles in disease transmission. The results in Chapters 2–4 are essentially well known results from the theory of branching processes that have been translated to the infectious disease context. This adaptation works because during the early stages of an outbreak, in a large population, the characteristics of growth in the number of infectives are similar to those of branching process population growth *and* it is the early stage of the outbreak that determines whether, or not, the outbreak takes off or fades out. These models tell us when a minor outbreak occurs and something about the nature of minor outbreaks, but are not able to tell us what happens beyond the early stages of a more substantial outbreak.

For convenience, the only public health intervention considered in Chapters 2, 3 and 4 is a mass immunization campaign with a vaccine that is fully protective. Ways to reflect the impact of other public health interventions in infectious disease models are built up in Chapters 5, 6 and 7. This needs a description of the way the infectiousness of an individual changes over time after being infected. Therefore Chapter 5 introduces a description of the dynamics of the infectivity of an infected individual over time. In Chapter 6 we explain how to model the impact of a vaccine that is only partially effective. Chapter 7 introduces a range of public health interventions based on social distancing and describes appropriate ways to incorporate these interventions into models.

When public health interventions are not adequate to prevent epidemics the focus changes to reducing the size of the epidemic. Chapter 8 looks at the effectiveness of interventions to reduce the size of an epidemic, while Chapter 9 studies the dynamics of case incidence of an epidemic over time and explains how different public health interventions affect these dynamics.

The use of modeling to provide insights into infectious disease control relies on observed numerical data in two important ways. The first is for estimating key model parameters. This is illustrated in a number of sections in Chapters 2 to 9. However, each of these illustrations of parameter estimation assumes that the chosen model provides an adequate description of the infection process. This highlights the second important use of data, namely its use to inform the choice of model. Chapter 10 gives illustrations of how data are used to inform model choice.

Exercises are included in each chapter. These are chosen to give the reader a good understanding of the concepts and results presented in the chapter.

The book aims for clarity by introducing concepts in simple settings. This means that results are not always presented in their most general form. Bibliographic notes are given at the end of chapters to point the reader to the literature where extensions and more general results may be found.

A glossary of terms and notation is given at the back of the book to assist readers.

1.4 Bibliographic notes

The little book on modeling epidemics by Farrington (2003) introduces several of the concepts used in this book. He assumes minimal mathematics and gives references to real world data.

CHAPTER 2

Minor outbreaks when infectives are homogeneous

Public health management of infectious diseases aims to prevent epidemics. It is therefore important to understand why some introduced infections lead to epidemics while others do not. In this chapter we identify a characteristic of transmission that indicates whether an epidemic is possible, or not. It is illustrated that this characteristic can be used to quantify public health intervention requirements capable of preventing epidemics.

The setting in this chapter is a large community in which every infected individual has the same potential to infect others.

2.1 When are outbreaks certain to be minor?

Suppose the large community is free from a specific infectious disease when a single newly-infected individual joins the community. Let π denote the probability that this introduction of the infection, by a lone infective, results in a *minor outbreak*. In Section 2.4 we describe in some detail what we mean by minor outbreak. For the moment let us simply think of it as an outbreak with very few eventual cases.

Our aim is to find an equation that can be solved for π. The derivation of this equation is made simple by assuming that the susceptible fraction does not change during the course of the outbreak, which is a reasonable approximation for a minor outbreak in a large community.

The outbreak is clearly minor if the primary infective infects no one. However, the primary infective can progress the outbreak by infecting j, say, community members. Then the outbreak can be minor only if each of the j transmission chains initiated by these j secondary infectives fades out quickly. As the community is large and infectives are homogeneous, each of the j secondary infectives initiates an independent transmission chain and each of these is a minor outbreak with probability π. This gives the equation

$$\pi = p_0 + p_1\pi + p_2\pi^2 + p_3\pi^3 + \cdots , \qquad (2.1)$$

where p_j is the probability that the primary infective infects a total of exactly j individuals during the course of his, or her, infectious period.

A study of solutions to Equation (2.1) gives our first important insight into the control of infectious diseases. Before stating this result it is useful to remind ourselves of the underlying assumptions and to introduce some terminology. The community is assumed to be large and infected individuals are assumed to be homogeneous, in the sense that each infective has the same potential to infect others. By the latter we mean that each infective can independently infect a random number of people, but the probability distribution of this random number is the same for each infective.

Each case arising from a contact between a given infective and a susceptible community member is an *offspring* of that infective. The probability distribution of the number infected by a single infective is called the *offspring distribution* and is given by probabilities $p_0, p_1, p_2, p_3, \cdots$. The mean number of offspring for each infective is

$$R = p_1 + 2p_2 + 3p_3 + \cdots . \tag{2.2}$$

We are now ready to state what we can learn from the solutions to Equation (2.1). The analysis given in Section 2.10.1 leads us to the

Transmission Threshold Property when infectives are homogeneous: *An outbreak arising from an imported infection is certain to be minor when* $R < 1$, *where* R *is given by (2.2).*

Worded another way, the threshold property says that an outbreak cannot take off if, *on average*, each infective replaces themselves by less than one infective. Expressed like this the property seems quite intuitive.

The key to the practical importance of the threshold property is that it tells us there is a single quantity, namely R, whose value indicates whether an epidemic can occur. The fact that R has a straightforward epidemiological interpretation, as the mean number of offspring produced by a single infective, strongly suggests that the threshold property is useful for planning public health measures capable of preventing epidemics. We now give our first illustration of this potential.

2.2 Preventing epidemics by mass immunization

To see how the threshold property informs strategies and requirements for the control of infectious diseases we need to understand how public health interventions can change R, the mean of the offspring distribution.

Consider a large community that is currently free from a certain infectious disease. Some community members may be immune to this infectious disease, from previous exposure to the infection. Assume that the current value of R for the disease in this community is greater than 1. In other words, the mean number of offspring for a primary infective of this infectious disease, should the infection be introduced into this community, has a value greater than 1.

Now suppose the community implements a mass vaccination campaign, with a vaccine that fully protects against infection, and the campaign is able to vaccinate a fraction v of community members. We say that the campaign achieves a *vaccination coverage* v. If individuals are selected for vaccination at random, the campaign fully immunizes a fraction v of all susceptible community members. It is assumed that the rate of interaction among community members is not altered by the immunization campaign.

The campaign changes the number of people an infective is likely to infect, because some contacted people are individuals who were susceptible before the campaign but are immune after the campaign. On average, a fraction v of contacts that would have led to infection pre-campaign does not lead to infection post-campaign. We deduce, heuristically, that R^*, the mean of the offspring distribution after the immunization campaign, is given by

$$R^* = (1 - v)R. \tag{2.3}$$

A more formal derivation of this result is given in Section 2.10.2.

From Equation (2.3) and the threshold property we deduce that after the immunization campaign there will only be minor outbreaks if $(1 - v)R < 1$. In other words, the immunization campaign should aim to achieve a vaccination coverage that is greater than

$$v^\dagger = 1 - 1/R, \tag{2.4}$$

because then only minor outbreaks can occur. We call $v^\dagger$ the *critical vaccination coverage*. It is the smallest fraction of community members that must be immunized to ensure an outbreak is minor.

Three sources of doubt about the practical public health value of this result for infectious disease control spring to mind. They are:

(i) the result depends on the value of R, which is usually unknown,
(ii) in practice individuals often differ in their potential to infect others,
(iii) it is not clear that the concept of *minor outbreak* used to deduce the result is suited to public health objectives.

To address the first concern we give methods to estimate R in Section 2.7, and later chapters. Chapters 3 and 4 give extensions of the transmission threshold property to community settings with a household structure and individuals of different type. Those extensions provide assurance about concern (ii). The third concern is allayed in Section 2.4, where we explore the properties of the concept of minor outbreak referred to in the threshold property.

Before attending to concerns (iii) it is useful to familiarize ourselves with the threshold parameter R.

2.3 Reproduction number

The concept of *reproduction number* plays a prominent role in discussions of infectious disease control. Its definition varies somewhat, depending on the community setting assumed and the type of model used to quantify it. For the setting of this chapter the definition of reproduction number is

$$\begin{aligned} R &= \text{mean number of individuals a single infective infects,} \\ &= \text{mean of the offspring distribution.} \end{aligned}$$

The name *reproduction number* stems from the fact that transmission models describe the reproductive dynamics of a population in which infectives are the individuals, infections are births and R describes the mean number of offspring (infections) an infective produces.

While the actual number of individuals infected by a given infective is integer-valued and random, the reproduction number R is a *mean* and is therefore non-random and usually not an integer. The mean of a probability distribution is usually thought of as a constant, but it is misleading to think of R as a constant. The offspring distribution for infectives of any given disease may differ between communities. Further, the offspring distribution changes over time during an epidemic and it may also change when a community responds to a public health intervention. As a consequence, the mean R varies across community settings and over the course of an epidemic. This warrants some discussion because, unfortunately, the way the term reproduction number is used in the literature is not consistent, which can lead to confusion.

Basic reproduction number

The *basic reproduction number*, denoted R_0, is a convenient place to start because it is defined for a more specific setting. Given a particular infectious disease, R_0 is the mean number of individuals a single infective infects in a large community in which every other individual is susceptible. The key requirements for a reproduction number to be R_0 are that there is no immunity present in the community and all individuals are interacting naturally. In particular, it is assumed there are no public health measures in place to curb transmission.

The numerical value of R_0 depends on the biology of the host-pathogen interaction. Specifically, R_0 depends on the way this interaction plays out in terms of the duration of the infectious period and the rate at which the infective sheds infectious agent during the infectious period. It also depends on the ease with which contacted susceptibles are able to ingest the infectious agent and the ease with which ingested pathogens settle within the host to multiply. These biological features make the numerical value of R_0 disease-specific. It is often reasonable to assume that these biological characteristics are similar for different communities.

The value of R_0 also depends on the number of individuals with which the infective makes contact and the nature of these contacts. These mixing characteristics make up the social component of R_0. In two culturally different communities the social elements affecting transmission of the infection may differ, which means that the value of R_0 for a specific disease may differ for these communities. For example, if shaking hands and kissing on the cheek are common ways of greeting in one community and greetings in the second community tend to consist of bowing, then the value of R_0 for these two communities may differ. The value of R_0 for two communities may also differ if their degree of crowding differs. Nevertheless, in practice differences in the value of R_0 between communities are usually not very large.

The actual value of the reproduction number at a given moment in time is rarely equal to R_0, because generally some community members have acquired immunity from previous exposure to the infection or from vaccination.

Effective reproduction number

The actual reproduction number, R, at a specified time in a given community is called the *effective reproduction number.* During the course of an epidemic R changes over time and it is sometimes useful to denote its value $R(t)$, where t is the time since the start of the epidemic. It is $R(0)$, the effective reproduction number at the start of the outbreak, that is key to consideration of requirements for the prevention of epidemics. In our discussion of prevention of epidemics, we refer to $R(0)$ as the *initial reproduction number.*

It is important not to confuse the basic reproduction number R_0 and the initial reproduction number $R(0)$. The basic reproduction number applies to a naive community, where all individuals are susceptible and no control measures are in place. The initial reproduction number is usually smaller than R_0, because it is adjusted for the presence of existing immunity and public health interventions present at the start of the outbreak. In the event of a newly emerged infection, such as Severe Acute Respiratory Syndrome (SARS) in 2002, we may have $R(0) = R_0$.

When social interaction is normal, i.e., not changed by public health measures or public response to health alerts, the initial reproduction number can be expressed in terms of the basic reproduction number by $R(0) = s_0 R_0$, where s_0 is the fraction of community members susceptible at the start of the outbreak. An individual's immunity may be from previous exposure to the infectious disease or vaccination.

Suppose now that the community is free of cases of the infectious disease when an immunization campaign is implemented, with a vaccine that is fully protective. Following the mass immunization campaign, with individuals selected for vaccination indiscriminately, the effective reproduction number at the start of a subsequent introduction of the infectious disease would be

$$R^*(0) \;=\; (1-v)s_0R_0,$$

where s_0 is the fraction of the community that was susceptible prior to the immunization campaign and v is the vaccination coverage achieved by the campaign. Post-campaign, minor outbreaks will be certain if the vaccination coverage v is greater than $v^\dagger = 1 - 1/(s_0R_0)$. These expressions for $R^*(0)$ and $v^\dagger$ are the same as Equations (2.3) and (2.4), merely written in a form that highlights the difference between the initial reproduction number and the basic reproduction number.

For notational convenience we will often suppress the time argument in $R(t)$ and simply use R to denote the effective reproduction number. In discussions about preventing epidemics R will be the initial reproduction number unless specified otherwise.

Mean trend in transmission

A concept of time is introduced, indirectly, by defining R as the mean number of offspring an infective has. It is not calendar time, but time measured in generations (of infectives). Consider an infectious disease that is freshly introduced. Generation 1 consists of the primary infectives who initiate the outbreak. All susceptibles who have an infectious contact with any of the primary infectives become the infectives of Generation 2. All susceptibles who avoid infectious contacts with Generation 1 infectives and have an infectious contact with a Generation 2 infective become the infectives of Generation 3, and so on. An example of the progress of transmission of the infection over the first six generations is shown in Figure 2.1.

Generation time is loosely related to calendar time, in a way that depends on characteristics of the infectious disease. Generations might overlap in calendar time because of variation in the time when an infective infects individuals.

Suppose now that Generation j consists of k infectives. Then the expected number of infectives in Generation $j+1$ is kR, because each infective has a mean number of R offspring. This tells us that the mean number of infectives is growing at the time of Generation j if R, the effective reproduction number of Generation j infectives, is greater than 1. The mean number of infectives is declining at the time of Generation j if $R < 1$.

This demonstrates that the effective R, at any "time," is the factor by which generation size tends to change as we go to the next generation.

It is this property of R that is the essence of definitions of reproduction number in more elaborate community settings, as we will see in Chapter 4.

We now address one of the sources of doubt mentioned in Section 2.2, on

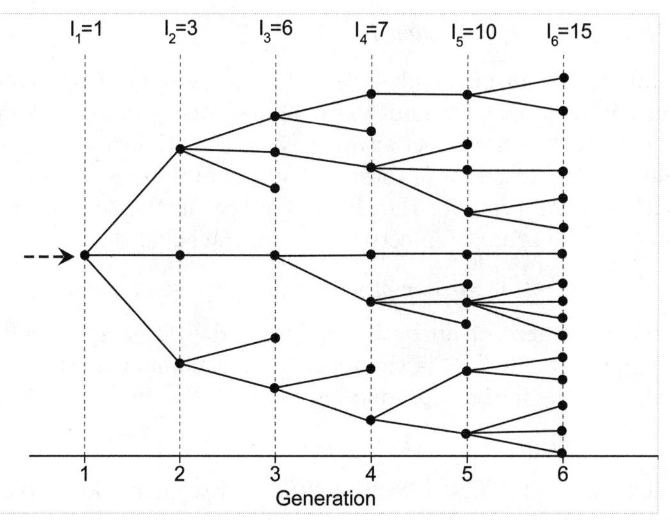

Figure 2.1 *Depiction of the transmission pattern and generations for an outbreak initiated by one external contact. The* $I_1, I_2, \ldots, I_6$ *shown at the top give the number of infectives in the first six generations.*

page 9, namely the concern about the practical relevance of the concept of minor outbreak referred to in the transmission threshold property.

2.4 What is a minor outbreak?

In public health, the definition of a minor outbreak is generally adapted to the severity of the disease associated with the infection. For example, an outbreak of Hendra virus* with five human cases would be considered a major outbreak, because the case-fatality rate in humans is about 60%. On the other hand, a substantially larger number of cases of the common cold would not be a cause for alarm.

The notion of minor outbreak used in this chapter was introduced mathematically, through Equation (2.1), for the probability of a minor outbreak. It has its roots in the theory of branching processes where the term "minor" is used to refer to "an outbreak of negligible size compared to an outbreak that expands without limit." That's not very helpful to us. To see if our notion of minor outbreak is useful for planning infectious disease control we take a look at the mean size of such an outbreak and the variation one might expect in the size of such outbreaks.

* Hendra virus can be transmitted from flying foxes, a natural resevoir for Hendra virus, to humans via horses.

2.4.1 *Mean outbreak size when* $R < 1$

The total size of an outbreak initiated when a single newly-infected individual joins a large community is 1, namely the primary case, when the initial infective does not infect anyone else. If the primary infective infects j community members, each of these j offspring initiates a separate independent outbreak. Allowing for the chance element in the number of offspring generated by the primary infective, we find the equation

$$\nu = 1 + p_1\nu + 2p_2\nu + 3p_3\nu + \cdots = 1 + \nu R$$

for ν, the mean size of an outbreak initiated by a single newly-infected primary infective. Here R is the reproduction number at the start of the outbreak, i.e., the initial reproduction number. Solving for ν gives

$$\nu = 1/(1 - R)\,, \qquad (2.5)$$

which holds when $0 \leq R < 1$. Section 2.10.3 gives a more detailed derivation of this equation.

From a practical point of view it is useful that the mean outbreak size is fully described by R. No other characteristics of the offspring distribution need to be known.

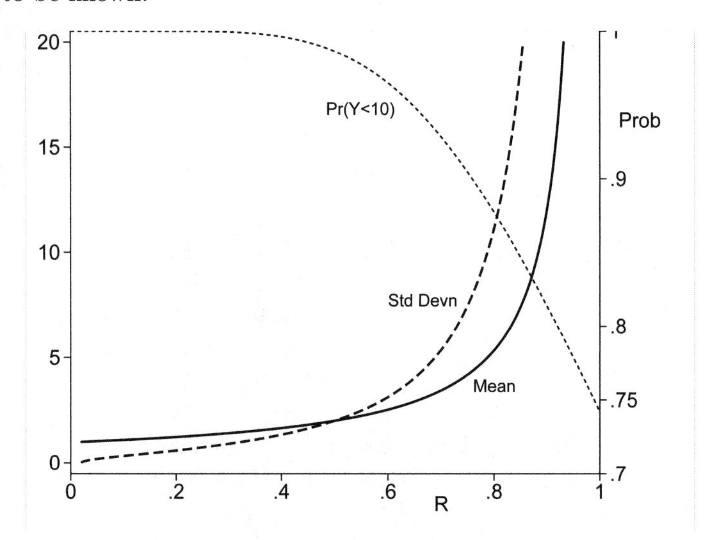

Figure 2.2 *Curves of*
(i) mean and standard deviation of total outbreak size (use left vertical axis), and
(ii) probability of less than 10 cases (use right vertical axis),
for different values of R, the mean of the offspring distribution.

The solid curve in Figure 2.2 shows the graph of the mean outbreak size, as in Equation (2.5), from which we note that

(i) it is small and increases slowly with R in the range $0 < R < 0.8$, and

(ii) it increases rapidly and becomes large in the range $0.9 < R < 1$.

This suggests that control efforts should aim to reduce the value of R to 0.8. As far as mean outbreak size is concerned, little is gained by reducing R further.

Minor outbreaks may also occur, by chance, when $R > 1$. However, the mean size is not given by Equation (2.5) for such minor outbreaks. The mean outbreak size when $R > 1$ is described in Section 2.10.4. Briefly, when $R > 1$ the mean outbreak size of a minor outbreak declines very quickly as R increases, as illustrated in Figure 2.9.

2.4.2 Variation in the size of a minor outbreak

The mean is only a partial reflection of the size of a minor outbreak, because chance can impact minor outbreaks substantially. To make public health decisions it helps to know how much variation occurs in the size of minor outbreaks.

One way to learn about variation is to look at the standard deviation of the total size of the outbreak. An argument similar to that which led to Equation (2.5) gives the standard deviation of the size of the outbreak as

$$\mathrm{SD}(Y) = \sigma/(1-R)^{3/2}, \quad \text{when} \quad 0 < R < 1, \tag{2.6}$$

where σ is the standard deviation of the offspring distribution. This result is derived in Section 2.10.3. We see that, whereas the mean outbreak size depends only on R, the variation in the outbreak size depends also on the variation in the number of individuals infected by a single infective.

The dashed curve in Figure 2.2 is the graph of the standard deviation $\mathrm{SD}(Y)$, as given by (2.6), under the assumption that the variance σ^2 is equal to the mean R. One distribution with this property is the Poisson distribution, a distribution that is often applied to data on counts of events over time. The Poisson distribution with mean R has probabilities given by

$$p_j = \frac{R^j\, \mathrm{e}^{-R}}{j!} \quad \text{for} \quad j = 0, 1, 2, 3, \ldots. \tag{2.7}$$

The dashed curve in Figure 2.2 indicates that the magnitude of the standard deviation of the outbreak size is of about the same order as its mean up to $R = 0.6$, but then becomes substantially larger than the mean. The Figure 2.2 graphs for ν and $\mathrm{SD}(Y)$ indicate that both the mean and the variability in outbreak size increase rapidly, and can become very large, as R approaches 1.

The standard deviation (2.6) is one way to indicate variation in the outbreak size and has the advantage of not assuming more about the offspring distribution than values of its mean and standard deviation. However, the values of the mean and standard deviation are influenced greatly by the right-hand tail of the distribution. Specifically, these measures can be large when the probability of a very large outbreak is small, but positive. It is therefore instructive, when making public health decisions about the control of outbreaks, to look also at the probability that the total outbreak size is less than 10, say.

2.4.3 Probability of fewer than 10 cases

The practical difficulty in making precise probability statements about the size of an outbreak is that we need to know the offspring distribution. That is, we need to know $p_0, p_1, p_2, p_3, \ldots$. This requires data that are difficult to collect. However, an illustrative computation is informative.

Suppose we would like to make a public health judgement about control on the basis of the probability of having less than 10 cases in total. To determine the probability that the outbreak size is less than 10 requires us to know $p_0, p_1, p_2, \ldots, p_7$ and p_8. For our illustration we assume the Poisson offspring distribution (2.7), which is a good working model in the infectious disease context. For this offspring distribution it can be shown, see for example Mott (1963), that Y, the size of an outbreak initiated by a single primary case, has the Borel-Tanner distribution given by

$$\Pr(Y = y) = \frac{1}{(y-1)!}\, y^{y-2} R^{y-1}\, \mathrm{e}^{-yR} \quad \text{for} \quad y = 1, 2, 3, \ldots . \tag{2.8}$$

Using this to compute $\Pr(Y < 10)$, for different values of R, gives the dotted curve in Figure 2.2. We see that $\Pr(Y < 10)$ is very close to 1 in the range $0 < R < 0.5$, but declines relatively quickly in the range $0.5 < R < 1$. However, $\Pr(Y < 10)$ remains above 0.8 up to $R = 0.92$ and equals 0.75 for $R = 0.99$. This paints a clearer picture of the possible scenarios than is given by looking only at the mean and standard deviation of the outbreak size. The large values of $\nu = 100$ and $\mathrm{SD}(Y) = 995$ for $R = 0.99$ are alarming, but less so when we also know that $\Pr(Y < 10) = 0.75$ for $R = 0.99$. This illustrates the dependence of the mean and standard deviation on the tail of the distribution and the value of looking at specific probabilities.

2.5 Probability of a minor outbreak

The probability of a minor outbreak tells us the risk that an epidemic will occur when the infectious disease is introduced. We have used the equation for this probability to show that a minor outbreak is certain when $R < 1$. There is also a chance, though no certainty, that a minor outbreak will occur when $R > 1$. The actual value of π, the probability of a minor outbreak, when $R > 1$, is also of public health interest. It is useful to know how its value is changed by specific public health interventions. For example, it would be useful to know that an intervention is able to increase the probability that an outbreak is minor by a substantial amount, such as raising its value to be close to 1 or increasing its value by a factor of two, or more.

Unfortunately neither the value of R, nor any other single quantity, determines the probability of a minor outbreak when $R > 1$. The solution to Equation (2.1) depends on the offspring distribution $p_0, p_1, p_2, \dots$ in a more complicated way when $R > 1$. Nevertheless, it is instructive to make illustrative calculations for a couple different offspring distributions. For these we choose the Poisson distribution and the Geometric distribution.

The Poisson distribution given by Equation (2.7) has mean R, variance R and its mode typically has a value near R. For this distribution Equation (2.1) can be written

$$\pi = e^{R(\pi-1)}, \tag{2.9}$$

which needs to be solved numerically for π.

For the Geometric distribution we use

$$p_j = \frac{1}{1+R}\left(\frac{R}{1+R}\right)^j, \qquad j = 0, 1, 2, 3, \dots, \tag{2.10}$$

because this form is parameterized in terms of R, the parameter of interest in the current context. This distribution has mean R and variance $R(1+R)$. It differs from the Poisson distribution by having a larger variance and having a mode that is zero irrespective of the value of R. Figure 2.3 shows the Poisson and Geometric distributions, each with mean $R = 3$.

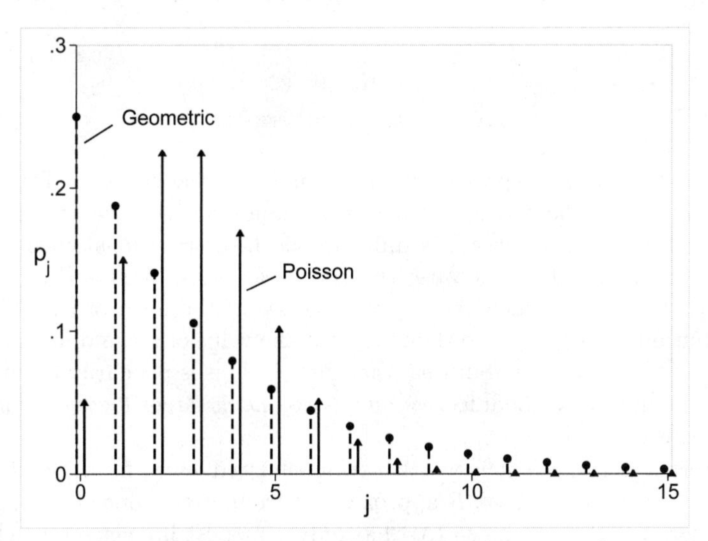

Figure 2.3 *Poisson and Geometric offspring distributions with mean $R = 3$.*

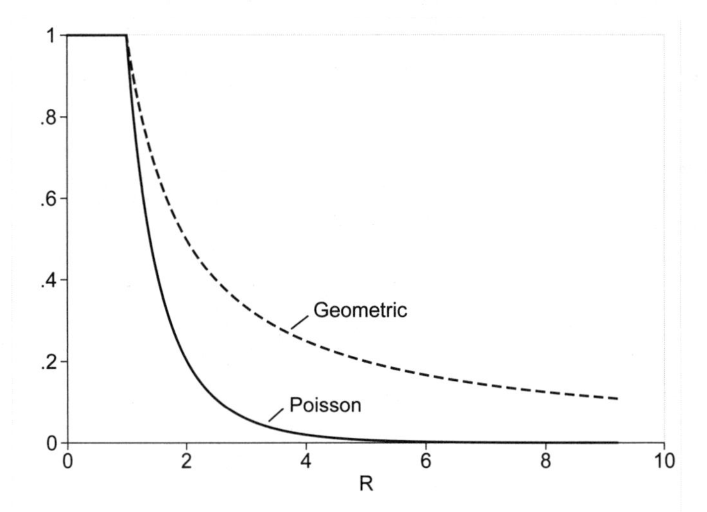

Figure 2.4 *The probability of a minor outbreak, π, for the Poisson and Geometric offspring distribution over a range of R values.*

For the Geometric distribution Equation (2.1) can be written

$$\pi = \frac{1}{1 + R - R\pi},$$

which has the convenience of an explicit solution, giving the probability of a minor outbreak as

$$\pi = \begin{cases} 1/R, & \text{if } R > 1, \\ 1, & \text{otherwise.} \end{cases} \tag{2.11}$$

Figure 2.4 shows the probability of a minor outbreak for each of these two offspring distributions over a range of R values. We see that π, the probability of a minor outbreak, is unity for both distributions when $R < 1$. That's as it should be, because the threshold property stated on page 8 tells us that $\pi = 1$ when $R < 1$, irrespective of the form of the offspring distribution. Figure 2.4 also shows us that the value of π can differ substantially for these two distributions when $R > 1$. This is primarily because p_0, the probability that the infective infects no one, is larger for the Geometric distribution.

In terms of control, it is worth noting that reducing the value of R has the greatest effect on π as R approaches 1 from above. Specifically, a 50% reduction in R from 8 down to 4 has only a modest impact on π, whereas a 50% reduction in R from 3 to 1.5 increases π substantially. Most realistic offspring distributions have this characteristic.

2.6 Importation of the infectious disease

Our discussion has assumed that the infectious disease is imported by a single newly-infected individual. That is, the primary case joined the community prior to the start of his infectious period. In practice importation can differ from this in numerous ways. We need to explore how different forms of importation affect the main results.

Primary infective arrives after the start of his infectious period

Consider how results change when the primary case acquired the infection outside the community and spent some of his infectious period outside the community before returning. The probability of a minor outbreak is then reduced from π as given by Equation (2.1) to

$$\pi' = p_0' + p_1'\pi + p_2'\pi^2 + p_3'\pi^3 + \cdots ,$$

where $p_0', p_1', p_2', p_3', \cdots$ is the distribution for the number of offspring produced in the community by the primary infective. With $\pi = 1$ the right-hand expression equals 1 and with $\pi < 1$ it is less than 1, unless $p_0' = 1$.

We conclude that the transmission threshold property given on page 8 remains true as stated.

In contrast, the expression for the mean of the outbreak size when $R < 1$ and the expression for the probability of a minor outbreak when $R > 1$ are changed. Specifically, the mean size of the outbreak when $R < 1$ is reduced to

$$\nu' = 1 + \frac{R'}{1 - R}, \tag{2.12}$$

where R', the mean number of community members infected by the primary infective after returning, is less than R.

The probability of a minor outbreak, when $R > 1$, is increased when the primary case spends part of his infectious period outside the community. The extent of this increase depends on the form of the offspring distributions.

Multiple introductions

Consider now how results change when the outbreak is initiated by the arrival of k newly infected individuals. Assuming that the introductory cases initiate chains of transmission independently, the probability of a minor outbreak is

$$\pi_k = \pi^k \quad \text{which is} \quad \begin{cases} = 1 & \text{when } \pi = 1, \\ = \pi & \text{when } \pi < 1 \text{ and } k = 1, \\ < \pi & \text{when } \pi < 1 \text{ and } k > 1. \end{cases}$$

It follows that again the threshold property given on page 8 holds as stated. However, when $R > 1$, the probability of a minor outbreak decreases rapidly as k, the number of primary cases, increases.

The mean size of the outbreak is

$$\nu_k = k/(1 - R)$$

when $R < 1$ and k newly-infected primary infectives initiate the outbreak. This assumes that each primary case independently initiates an outbreak.

2.7 Estimating R

The current effective reproduction number R plays a key role in determining public health interventions capable of preventing epidemics. It is therefore important to know its value for a given infectious disease in our community. We therefore need ways to estimate R. Methods for estimating R depend on (i) the type of data available, and
(ii) a model that is appropriate for the available data.

In this section we illustrate ways to estimate R. The data sets used in these illustrations are ones for which the simple models of this chapter are appropriate.

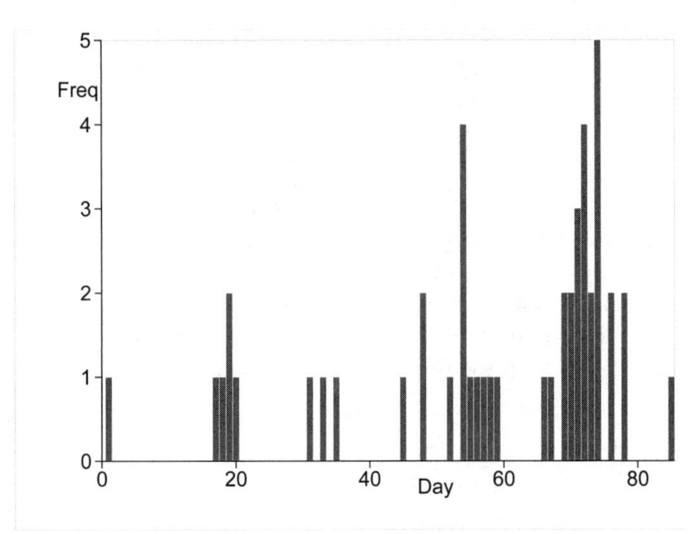

Figure 2.5 *Early-stage incidence of smallpox in the São Paulo epidemic of 1956.*

2.7.1 Data on case clusters

The latent period of an infectious disease is the period from infection until the infected person becomes infectious. Some infectious diseases, including chicken pox, measles and smallpox, have a relatively long latent period. For such diseases cases tend to be clustered in time during the early stage of an outbreak. This is illustrated by the incidence data for variola minor, the milder form of smallpox, shown in Figure 2.5. These data, presented by Rodrigues-da-Silva et al. (1963), are for the early cases of the 1956 epidemic in Vila Guarani, a semi-isolated workers' residential district of São Paulo city, Brazil. The initial local case, infected by one of two infected travelers who passed through, had onset of symptoms on April 9, 1956 (Day 1 in Figure 2.5). This is the sole case of Generation 1. The subsequent clusters of cases are the generations of the population process for infectives. Specifically, the initial case produced five offspring, who had onset of symptoms on days 17 to 20. They are the cases of Generation 2. These five cases produced Generation 3, consisting of the three cases with onset on days 31 to 35. In this way we deduce the realized values of the generation sizes I_1, I_2, I_3, I_4 and I_5 shown in Table 2.1.

Table 2.1: *Generations of variola minor cases*

Generation, j	1	2	3	4	5
Cases, I_j	1	5	3	12	24

As R is the mean of the offspring distribution, the sample mean is a natural estimate of R. Each generation consists of the offspring of the previous generation, so we have $I_1 + I_2 + I_3 + I_4 = 21$ parents giving rise to $I_2 + I_3 + I_4 + I_5 = 44$ offspring. Therefore, in this context, $44/21$ is the sample mean, which gives the estimate $\widehat{R} = 2.10$ for the initial reproduction number R. Section 2.10.5 introduces this estimate more formally.

The basic reproduction number for smallpox is thought to fall in the range of 3.5–6. The smaller estimate $\widehat{R} = 2.10$ suggests that there was some immunity in this population due to earlier exposure to smallpox or vaccination. The value $1 - 1/\widehat{R} = 0.52$ suggests that if at least 52% of the community's susceptibles had been immunized prior to this epidemic, then this introduction of the infection would have led to a minor outbreak with probability 1.

An estimate should always be accompanied by a measure of its precision. By analogy with well-known results for the sample mean we propose

$$\text{s.e.}(\widehat{R}) \;=\; \widehat{\sigma}/\sqrt{I_1 + I_2 + I_3 + I_4} \;=\; \widehat{\sigma}/\sqrt{21}\,,$$

as the standard error for this estimate, where $\widehat{\sigma}$ is an estimate of σ, the standard deviation of the offspring distribution. One way to estimate σ is to assume a form for the offspring distribution. For example, assuming a Poisson offspring distribution gives the estimate $\widehat{\sigma} = \sqrt{\widehat{R}} = 1.45$ and a standard error $\text{s.e.}(\widehat{R}) = 0.32$, while a Geometric offspring distribution gives the estimate $\widehat{\sigma} = \sqrt{\widehat{R}(1+\widehat{R})} = 2.55$ and a standard error s.e.$(\widehat{R}) = 0.56$. In Section 2.10.5 we estimate σ by a method that does not assume a specific type of offspring distribution. It leads to the standard error s.e.$(\widehat{R}) = 0.60$.

There are two main reasons why we used only data on the first five generations in this application. Firstly, widespread vaccination was introduced in response to the increasing number of cases over the first five generations and behavior is also likely to have changed. Such responses change the value of the reproduction number, and our aim was to estimate the initial reproduction number R. Secondly, the natural variation in infection times of cases leads to an overlap in later generations, making generation counts beyond generation five unreliable. For this method of estimation there is also a concern that as case numbers increase the effective reproduction number becomes smaller because the fraction of individuals who are susceptible decreases as more individuals are infected.

2.7.2 Data on the size of minor outbreaks

The State of Victoria, Australia, has a long history of vaccinating against measles, including a two-dose schedule targeting children aged 12 months and 5 years. The coverage achieved in these doses was adequate to interrupt endemic transmission of measles regularly. Additional to the two-dose schedule, in 1998 there was an Australia-wide Measles Control Campaign that aimed to vaccinate all primary schoolchildren, aged 5–12 years, with a dose of measles-mumps-rubella vaccine. The rapid reduction of the susceptible fraction from such a vaccination campaign was hoped to keep the reproduction number below the threshold value of one for some time, because replenishment of the susceptible pool by births and immigration takes time. However, minor outbreaks recur because widespread travel and endemic transmission of the disease in other regions mean that re-introductions are likely.

To assess the effectiveness of the measles control campaign and to monitor the value of R over time, measles surveillance was enhanced and outbreaks were investigated over the period 1998 to mid-2003. Table 2.2 gives the frequency distribution for the sizes of 39 outbreaks of measles observed during this period. Each of these outbreaks had one primary case. Our aim is to use these data to estimate R.

Table 2.2: *Sizes of 39 measles outbreaks, Victoria 1998–2003*

Outbreak size	1	2	3	4	5	6	15	18	20	51	75
Observed frequency	22	6	2	2	1	1	1	1	1	1	1

Each single outbreak contains little information, but together they provide useful information about R. A quick and easy estimate of R is obtained by noting that there is a total of 238 cases in these 39 outbreaks. The 39 introductory cases of these outbreaks were infected by an external contact. Therefore, 238 infectives have generated 199 offspring within the community, which means that an infective had an average of $199/238 = 0.836$ offspring. This is a natural estimate of R, but this method of estimating the effective reproduction number does not suggest a convenient way to provide a standard error for the estimate. We therefore describe two other approaches for estimating R. They give the same estimate, but have the advantage of also providing a standard error.

For the first approach we view the sizes of the 39 outbreaks as observations on independent random variables $Y_1, Y_2, Y_3, \ldots, Y_{39}$. Using (2.5), each Y_j has mean $1/(1-R)$. Therefore the sample mean of these outbreak sizes, $\bar{y} = 6.10$, is a natural estimate of $1/(1-R)$. This leads to the estimate $\widehat{R} = 0.836$ of R. The sample standard deviation of the 39 outbreak sizes is 14.40, so that $\text{s.e.}(\bar{y}) = 14.40/\sqrt{39} = 2.306$. Use of the Delta Method, see Section 2.10.6, gives the standard error $\text{s.e.}(\widehat{R}) = \text{s.e.}(\bar{y})/\bar{y}^2 = 0.062$.

Another way to estimate R is to assume a specific form for the offspring distribution and use maximum likelihood estimation. For example, when we assume a Poisson offspring distribution the maximum likelihood estimate turns out to be the same as the estimate $\widehat{R} = 0.836$ found above. Large-sample likelihood methods give an associated standard error of 0.059, which is similar to the 0.062 reported above; see Section 2.10.6 for details.

The main motivation for estimating R from such data is to check that its value lies adequately below 1. Such monitoring of the value of R might include expressing R as $\alpha + \beta t$, where t denotes the calendar time of the outbreak. Using data on the outbreak sizes we can estimate the parameters α and β. This allows us to check whether R might be increasing over time, perhaps due to an increase in the proportion of susceptibles in the population, as a result of waning immunity in individuals or an inadequate vaccination schedule for recently born infants.

2.8 Discussion

The minor-major outbreak dichotomy

Our discussion of minor outbreaks has implicitly used the fact that an outbreak will be either minor or become an epidemic. Having introduced basic modeling concepts, such as generations of infectives and offspring distributions, we are now able to illustrate this dichotomy of outbreaks by simulation.

Assume that an outbreak is initiated by a single infective in a community with 1000 susceptible individuals. Take the offspring distribution to be Poisson, initially with mean 1.5. That is, the initial reproduction number is $R = 1.5$. The depletion of susceptibles is allowed for by adjusting the mean of the offspring distribution for a given generation in a way that acknowledges the immunity acquired by infectives of previous generations. For each infective of a given generation the mean number of offspring is $1.5 \times (1000 - x)/1000$, where x is the total number of infectives realized in previous generations.

The sizes of 10,000 outbreaks simulated in this way are summarized by the histogram of Figure 2.6. The dichotomy in the realized outbreak sizes is clearly visible. The total number of cases was less than 20 for a substantial number of outbreaks. The outbreak size was between 450 and 750 for nearly all other outbreaks. The number of outbreak sizes outside these two ranges is negligible, which illustrates why it makes sense to talk about a minor outbreak occurring with probability π and a major outbreak, or epidemic, occurring with probability $1 - \pi$.

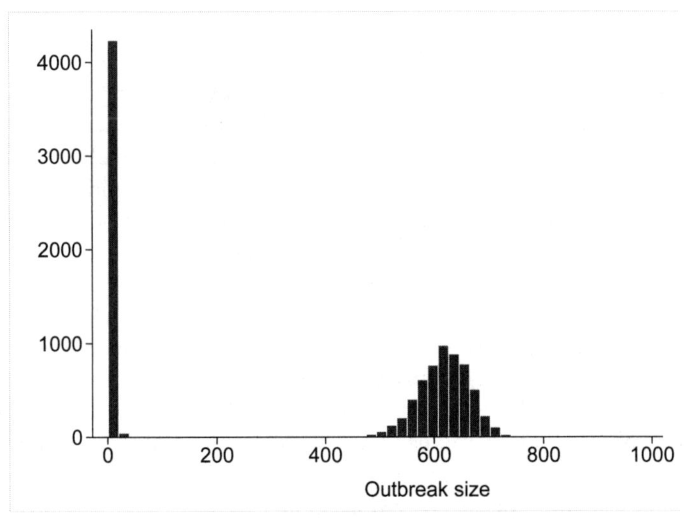

Figure 2.6 *Histogram for 10,000 simulated outbreak sizes in a community of 1000 susceptibles, where each outbreak is initiated by a single primary infective and the offspring distribution is Poisson. The mean number of offspring is initially 1.5 and is subsequently adjusted, following each generation, to be proportional to the fraction of community members still susceptible.*

To summarize the full range of results for the 10,000 simulations in one graph we had to use a large bin width for the histogram in Figure 2.6. By doing so we lose some detail. In Figure 2.7, Graph A (the graph on the left) shows the relative frequencies of the sizes of the minor outbreaks of Figure 2.6 using a scale for the horizontal axis that is better suited to display the frequencies for minor outbreaks. For comparison Graph B of Figure 2.7 shows the probabilities for the Borel-Tanner distribution (2.8) that corresponds to this setting. The latter distribution applies when we ignore the depletion of susceptibles. The agreement is seen to be good, illustrating that depletion in susceptibles affects the outcome of a minor outbreak only minimally.

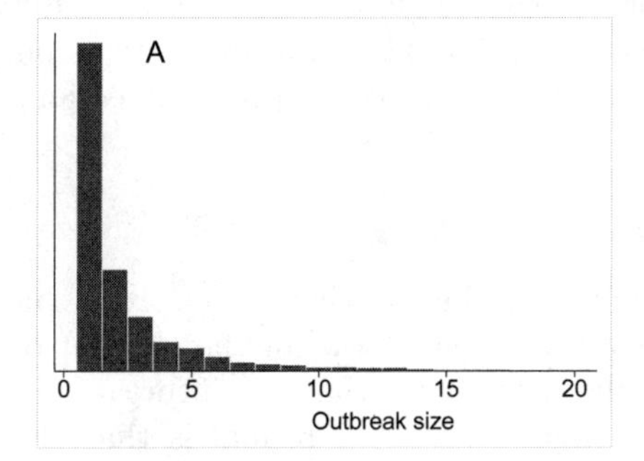

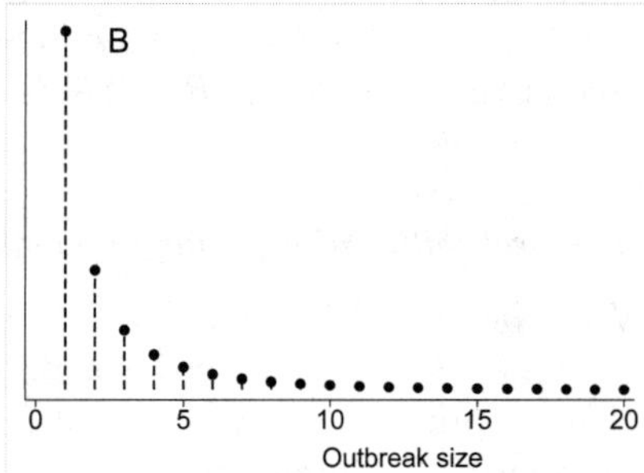

Figure 2.7 *Graph A shows the relative frequencies of the minor outbreaks in Figure 2.6 using a more suitable scale for the horizontal axis. Graph B shows the probabilities of the corresponding Borel-Tanner distribution.*

The transmission threshold property

The transmission threshold property is the main modeling tool for guiding public health interventions aimed at preventing epidemics. Its name reflects the fact that R, which is a measure of the rate of transmission, has a threshold value. The value $R = 1$ is a threshold value because outbreaks initiated when $R > 1$ can be dramatically different from the minor outbreaks that are sure to occur when $R < 1$.

The larger part of the literature concerned with infectious disease modeling uses deterministic models. That is, they ignore the chance component of transmission altogether. Although the transmission threshold property on page 8 is stated in terms of probability, deterministic models can capture the main part of this property. We can see this from the following crude argument. If each infective generates exactly two new infections, then sizes of the early generations of an outbreak with one primary case will be 1, 2, 4, 8, 16, 32, 64 and 128. That is, generation size increases and does so rapidly. Now suppose each infective generates R new infections, where we allow R to take non-integer values to reflect the average number of new infections. The progression of the generation sizes is then 1, R, R^2, R^3, $R^4, \cdots$. Such a series increases rapidly when $R > 1$ and decreases rapidly when $R < 1$. This indicates that the early growth of the outbreak when $R > 1$ differs markedly from what its early growth would be if $R < 1$. Like the stochastic version, this overly simple deterministic model indicates that much is to be gained by a public health intervention that is able to reduce R to a value below 1.

It is important to understand the concept of a minor outbreak as used in the statement of the transmission threshold property. Specifically, we must understand that such a "minor outbreak" can be quite large when R is only just below 1. Results like those in Sections 2.4 and 2.5 indicate that a good rule of thumb is to set $R \leq 0.8$ as a target for the control of an infectious disease.

The probability of a minor outbreak when $R > 1$

What deterministic models fail to capture is the fact that an outbreak can be minor when $R > 1$. Stochastic models, which allow for the element of chance, provide a way to quantify the probability that an outbreak will be minor. An interesting aspect to come out of our results is that the probability of a minor outbreak can be large even though $R > 1$; see Figure 2.4. An extreme example of this occurs when an infective infects either no one, with probability 0.99, or 200 individuals, with probability 0.01. For this offspring distribution the mean is $R = 2$ indicating that an epidemic is possible, but the probability of a minor outbreak resulting from one primary case is at least 0.99, because that is the probability of the initial infective infecting no one. This is not a real-world example, but it does make the point that decisions about infectious disease control measures should not be based solely on the expected size of a potential epidemic. When $R > 1$, the probability that an epidemic does not occur can also have a role to play in transmission management.

Practical value of the results

The homogeneity of infectives assumed in this chapter is not strictly true in real community settings. Nevertheless predictions of the likely outcome of a newly introduced infection obtained under this assumption are good enough to be of practical value. Two facts support this claim. First, the key results reported in this chapter are robust against moderate deviation from the assumed homogeneity because transmission of infection is first and foremost driven by reproduction of infectives and reproduction is precisely the feature on which our model is based. Second, in the next two chapters we obtain analogous results for settings that allow heterogeneity.

The quantitative description provided by our simple model assists us by:

(i) indicating the likely outcomes when an infectious disease is newly introduced and how different interventions will alter these outcomes,

(ii) providing the potential for a timely assessment of the intervention requirements for the prevention of an epidemic, and

(iii) enabling us to identify the data needed to inform the response to an outbreak of a newly emerged infection.

Application of the transmission threshold property, and other results, to inform the response to an outbreak of a newly emerged infection requires data to estimate R, the initial reproduction number. Part of a preparedness plan should therefore include preparedness to collect data that enable timely estimation of R. In the absence of data from previous outbreaks it is necessary to estimate R from data observed during the initial stage of the outbreak of the newly introduced infection. Data requests made during the early stage of an outbreak should preferably be minimal in extent. Then the data can be made available rapidly and their collection does not interfere unnecessarily with the urgent tasks of treating patients and implementing public health interventions to mitigate transmission. To enable an early assessment of the effort required to prevent an epidemic of a newly emerged infectious disease, such a scant data set might consist of timely reports of daily incidence for the first 100 cases and about 20 observations on the serial interval. The serial interval is the duration of time between onset of clinical symptoms in an infective and symptom onset in one of his offspring.

2.9 Exercises

1. Suppose each infective independently infects 0, 1 or 2 individuals with probability 0.2, 0.3 and 0.5, respectively.

   (a) Find R, the mean of the offspring distribution. What does its value tell you about the probability of a minor outbreak?

   (b) Find the solutions to Equation (2.1), namely

   $$x = p_0 + p_1 x + p_2 x^2 + p_3 x^3 + \cdots ,$$

   for this offspring distribution.

   (c) Deduce the value of π, the probability of a minor outbreak, for this offspring distribution.

2. Assume a Poisson offspring distribution. Then π, the probability of a minor outbreak, is given by a solution of Equation (2.9), namely

   $$\pi = \mathrm{e}^{R(\pi-1)}.$$

   (a) Express R as a function of π.

   (b) Explain how the expression found in (a) can be used, with the aid of a spreadsheet, to obtain the solid-line graph of Figure 2.4.

3. A certain disease has basic reproduction number 5 in a community with all members susceptible. A vaccine becomes available which provides complete immunity 90% of the time and fails 10% of the time. The vaccinee remains completely susceptible when his vaccination fails.

What fraction of community members must be vaccinated to prevent epidemics?

4. A certain disease has basic reproduction number 5 in a community with all members susceptible. In a mass immunization campaign, with a very effective vaccine, a coverage of v is achieved. Being dissatisfied with the coverage achieved, a second immunization campaign is administered a short time later. Community members are included in the second campaign independently of whether they were vaccinated during the first campaign or not. The second campaign also achieves a coverage of v.

   Determine the smallest value of v that prevents epidemics with this two-dose strategy.

5. An infectious disease is introduced into a large community and results in an epidemic during which 25% of community members are infected.

   What can be said about the value of the effective reproduction number

   (a) at the start of the epidemic, and
   (b) at the end of the epidemic?

   Give reasons for your answers.

6. Consider an initial reproduction number R and let $R' = \sqrt{R}$.

   Explain why the statement of the transmission threshold property, on page 8, remains true when R is replaced by R'.

7. The long latent period of measles makes it possible to allocate cases of the minor outbreaks of Table 2.2 into generations. Consider the following two extremes of such an allocation:

   Scenario 1. Every secondary case was infected by the primary infective. This implies that secondary infectives infected no one.
   Scenario 2. Each infective infects either 0 or 1 individual.

   (a) For each of these two scenarios

      (i) determine the number of generations each outbreak endured,
      (ii) give the observed frequency distribution for the number of offspring generated by infectives, and
      (iii) use the observed frequency distribution to estimate the mean of the offspring distribution.

   (b) How does the estimate of R change by knowing the number of offspring for each infective?

8. *Preparedness for an outbreak and timely response.*
   Suppose a newly emerged infectious disease has an initial reproduction number of 5 in a large community. A complete range of available public health interventions can reduce the reproduction number to 0.8. The time needed to initiate these interventions depends on how well the

community has prepared itself for a response to an emerging infectious disease. Suppose that the infectious disease is introduced by one newly infected individual and the first generation for which the full range of interventions can mitigate transmission of the infection is generation k.

(a) Compute ν_k, the mean outbreak size, when

(i) $k = 1$, i.e., right from the start,

(ii) $k = 2$, and

(iii) $k = 4$.

Assume the reproduction number is 5 in earlier generations.

(b) Comment on the consequences of delay in the introduction of public health interventions.

9. Suppose the number of susceptibles infected by an infective who spends his entire infectious period within the community has a Geometric distribution with mean R, as given by Equation (2.10).
Assume that an outbreak is initiated by a lone introductory infective who enters the community after the start of his infectious period. More specifically, assume that the number of community members the introductory case infects during the remainder of his infectious period has a Geometric distribution with mean $\frac{1}{2}R$.

(a) Find an expression for π', the probability that the outbreak is minor.

(b) Graphically, or otherwise, compare π' with π, the probability that the outbreak would be minor had the primary infective entered the community prior to the start of his infectious period.

10. Suppose a community is currently free from a certain infectious disease and that its initial reproduction number is 2 when a community member, A say, is infected while visiting relatives abroad. Assume that individual A returns home after the start of his infectious period, so that the mean number of individuals he infects in his community is $2f$, where $0 \leq f \leq 1$.

Sketch the graph of π, the probability that the return of individual A results in a minor outbreak, against f under the assumption that the offspring distribution is Geometric for every infective.

11. In 1971 countries in Europe were considering whether to abandon vaccination against smallpox. One aspect looked at by participants in the debate was the frequency and size of smallpox outbreaks over the recent past. In the preceding decade there had been 28 outbreaks, which resulted in a total of 391 cases of smallpox; see World Health Organization (1971a, b). Assume that each outbreak was initiated by one primary infective and suppose that the basic reproduction number of smallpox was estimated, from earlier data, to be 4.2.

(a) Give an estimate of θ, the fraction of the community that was immune over the preceding decade.

(b) Estimate θ by an approximate 95% confidence interval, assuming a Poisson offspring distribution.
[Hint: The mean and variance of the Borel-Tanner distribution given by (2.8) are $1/(1-R)$ and $R/(1-R)^3$, respectively.]

12. Use the argument given in Section 2.10.3 to derive Equation (2.12).

13. In a branching process model for the number of individuals in a population an offspring is a birth generated by an individual, i.e., a fresh individual. In the infectious disease context an offspring is a new infection, i.e., a susceptible who becomes an infective. This differs from the branching process offspring in that two or more individuals could have an infectious contact with the same susceptible individual.

    Explain why, despite this difference, we are able to adapt a major result of branching processes to arrive at the transmission threshold property.

2.10 Supplementary material

2.10.1 Transmission threshold

To learn about π, the probability of a minor outbreak, we first express Equation (2.1) as

$$x = g(x), \qquad \text{for } x \geq 0, \tag{2.13}$$

where $g(x) = \sum_{j=0}^{\infty} p_j x^j$ is the probability generating function of the offspring distribution. To cover all possible offspring distributions only the requirements $p_j \geq 0$ for $j = 0, 1, 2, \ldots$ and $\sum_{j=0}^{\infty} p_j = 1$ are imposed. Note that $x = 1$ is always a solution, because $g(1) = \sum_{j=0}^{\infty} p_j = 1$. However π is not necessarily 1, because Equation (2.13) might have more than one solution.

All solutions of (2.13) are given by the points of intersection of the curve $y = g(x)$ with the straight line $y = x$. Our interest is in solutions in the domain $0 \leq x \leq 1$, because π is a probability.

First consider an offspring distribution with $p_0 + p_1 = 1$ and $p_1 < 1$. Then both $y = x$ and $y = g(x) = p_0 + p_1 x$ are straight lines and their only point of intersection occurs at $x = 1$. Hence $\pi = 1$ in this case, which makes sense because the number of infectives cannot increase for such an offspring distribution.

Now suppose $p_0 + p_1 < 1$. Then the second derivative of $g(x)$, namely $g''(x) = \sum_{j=2} j(j-1)p_j x^{j-2}$, is positive for all $x > 0$. Therefore $g(x)$ is a convex function, like each of the three illustrative curves shown in Figure 2.8. This means the curve $y = g(x)$ can intersect the straight line $y = x$ at most twice. One point of intersection occurs at $x = 1$. The location of the other point of intersection, if any, is determined by the value of $g'(1)$, the gradient of $y = g(x)$ at $x = 1$.

The solution $x = 1$ is the only solution of Equation (2.13) when $g'(1) = 1$,

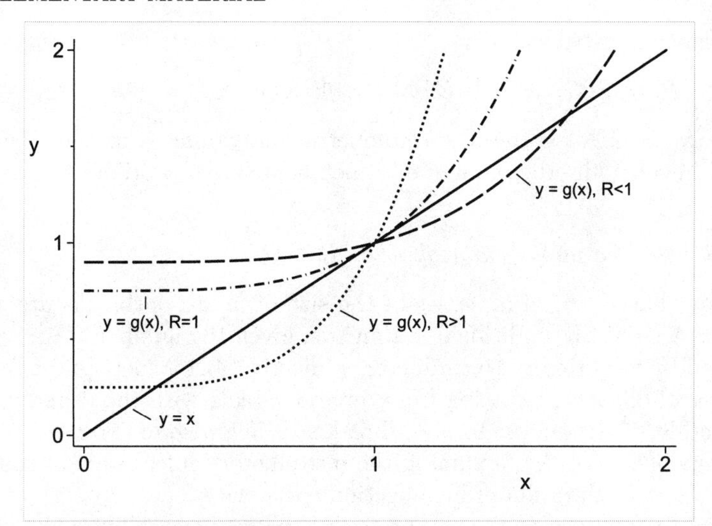

Figure 2.8 *Graphs of three probability generating functions $g(x)$. Solutions of Equation (2.13) occur where $y = g(x)$ intersects the straight line $y = x$. The smallest x value among intersection points gives π, the probability of a minor outbreak.*

because then the line $y = x$ is tangential to the curve $y = g(x)$ at $x = 1$. Therefore $\pi = 1$ also in this case.

When the gradient $g'(1)$ is less than 1 there is a second solution for some value of x greater than 1, so again $\pi = 1$.

Finally, when the gradient $g'(1)$ is greater than 1 there is a second solution for some value of x less than 1 and this is the value of π. Its actual value depends on the particular offspring distribution.

The threshold property stated on page 8 follows by observing that the gradient $g'(1) = \sum_{j=1} jp_j = R$, the mean number of individuals infected by a single infective.

2.10.2 *Effect of immunity on the mean of the offspring distribution*

Assume the community is large and close contacts are made independently. Define an *infectious contact* between two individuals as a contact that is sufficiently close to transmit the infection if the two individuals consist of one susceptible and one infectious person. Suppose the fraction of immune individuals is v and the remaining individuals are fully susceptible.

In such a partially immune community an infected individual who makes X infectious contacts infects Z individuals, where the conditional distribution of Z, given $X = x$, is Binomial$(x, 1 - v)$. The unconditional mean of the offspring distribution is

$$R = \mathrm{E}(Z) = \mathrm{E}[\mathrm{E}(Z \mid X)] = \mathrm{E}[X(1-v)] = (1-v)R_0,$$

where $R_0 = \mathrm{E}(X)$ is the mean number of individuals a primary infective would infect if all other community members are susceptible.

2.10.3 Size of a minor outbreak when $R < 1$

Assume that $R < 1$. Properties of the size of minor outbreaks are conveniently derived by conditional arguments, given the number of individuals infected by the primary (introductory) infective. Let X denote the random number of offspring resulting from direct contacts with the primary infective and let Y denote the total outbreak size. We wish to express $\nu = \mathrm{E}(Y)$ in terms of $R = \mathrm{E}(X)$, assuming the introductory infective is in the community for the duration of his infectious period.

Conditionally, given $X = x$, the size of the outbreak Y may be written

$$Y = \begin{cases} 1, & \text{if } x = 0, \\ 1 + Y_1 + \cdots + Y_x, & \text{if } x > 0, \end{cases} \tag{2.14}$$

where $Y_1, Y_2, \ldots, Y_x$ are independently distributed random variables with the same distribution as Y.

Mean outbreak size

Using (2.14) we find

$$\begin{aligned} \mathrm{E}(Y \mid X = x) &= \begin{cases} 1, & \text{if } x = 0, \\ 1 + \mathrm{E}(Y_1) + \mathrm{E}(Y_2) + \cdots + \mathrm{E}(Y_x), & \text{if } x > 0, \end{cases} \\ &= 1 + x\mathrm{E}(Y). \end{aligned}$$

Therefore, provided $R < 1$,

$$\mathrm{E}(Y) = \mathrm{E}[\mathrm{E}(Y \mid X)] = \mathrm{E}[1 + X\mathrm{E}(Y)] = 1 + \mathrm{E}(X)\mathrm{E}(Y).$$

Solving for $\mathrm{E}(Y)$ gives $\nu = 1/(1-R)$, as in Equation (2.5), where $R = \mathrm{E}(X)$ is the reproduction number at the start of the outbreak.

Standard deviation of outbreak size

Using (2.14) again we find

$$\mathrm{Var}(Y \mid X = x) = x\,\mathrm{Var}(Y).$$

This leads to

$$\mathrm{Var}(Y) = \mathrm{E}[\mathrm{Var}(Y \mid X)] + \mathrm{Var}[\mathrm{E}(Y \mid X)] = \mathrm{E}(X)\mathrm{Var}(Y) + [\mathrm{E}(Y)]^2\mathrm{Var}(X).$$

Substituting $\mathrm{E}(X) = R$, $\mathrm{Var}(X) = \sigma^2$ and $\mathrm{E}(Y) = 1/(1-R)$ gives the standard deviation

$$\mathrm{SD}(Y) \;=\; \sigma/(1-R)^{3/2}, \quad \text{when} \quad 0 < R < 1.$$

2.10.4 Size of a minor outbreak when $R > 1$

Consider an infectious disease for which $R > 1$ in a certain large community. We have seen that, although less than 1, the probability of a minor outbreak can be large when $R > 1$. It is therefore of interest to quantify the size of minor outbreaks that occur when $R > 1$.

For this infectious disease we look at outbreaks initiated by a single newly infected individual. Suppose the offspring distribution has probability generating function

$$g(x) \;=\; p_0 + p_1 x + p_2 x^2 + p_3 x^3 + \cdots, \qquad x \geq 0.$$

The infectious disease transmission process, conditional on a minor outbreak occurring, behaves like a transmission process in which infectives have an offspring distribution with probability generating function $g_{\mathrm{C}}(x) = \frac{1}{\pi} g(\pi x)$; see Waugh (1958). This does not change the process when $R < 1$, because then $\pi = 1$. That's as it should be. On the other hand, when $R > 1$ the process changes. Specifically, the mean of the offspring distribution then becomes $R_{\mathrm{C}} = g'_{\mathrm{C}}(1) = g'(\pi)$ and the mean total size of a minor outbreak initiated by a single newly infected community member is $1/(1-R_{\mathrm{C}})$. The value of R_{C} depends on the form of the unconditional offspring distribution. For example, the Poisson distribution has probability generating function $g(x) = \mathrm{e}^{R(x-1)}$, which gives $R_{\mathrm{C}} = \pi R$ as the mean number of offspring an infective has in a minor outbreak. On the other hand, the Geometric distribution has probability generation function $g(x) = 1/(1 + R - Rx)$, which gives $R_{\mathrm{C}} = \pi^2 R$.

We have $\pi = 1$ when $R < 1$, giving $R_{\mathrm{C}} = R$ and a mean outbreak size of $1/(1-R)$ for both offspring distributions, in agreement with the results of Section 2.4.1.

Figure 2.9 shows the graphs of $1/(1-R_{\mathrm{C}})$, the mean of the total outbreak size among all outbreaks that are minor, when the underlining offspring distribution is Poisson and Geometric for a range of values of R. The curves are identical over the range $0 < R < 1$, because the mean outbreak size is not distribution-dependent over that range. The curves differ over the range $R > 1$, but the difference is seen to be small. The very rapid drop in the mean outbreak size as R increases from 1 is noteworthy. It suggests strongly that when $R > 2$ a minor outbreak will occur only if, due to chance, the first few infectives have very few offspring causing the outbreak to fade out almost immediately.

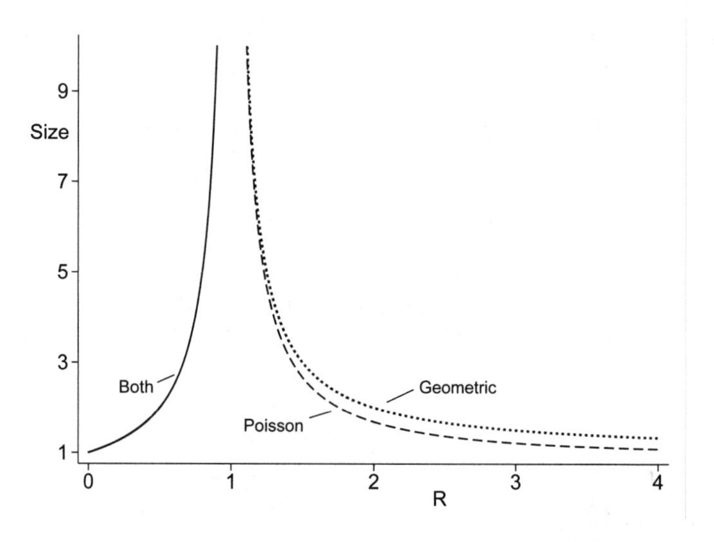

Figure 2.9 *Mean outbreak size, conditional on a minor outbreak, for the Poisson and Geometric offspring distributions with mean R.*

2.10.5 Estimating R from case clusters at the start of an epidemic

Suppose we have data on generation sizes $I_1, I_2, \dots, I_k$ for an outbreak initiated by the I_1 cases of Generation 1. Then each of I_j/I_{j-1}, $j = 2, 3, \dots, k$, is a sample mean, because I_j is the total number of offspring produced by I_{j-1} parents. These $k-1$ unbiased estimators for R can be pooled to provide a single, more efficient estimator for R. One way of doing this is to take their weighted average $\sum_{j=2}^{k} W_j(I_j/I_{j-1})$, where the weights W_j sum to unity. For such linear combinations of unbiased estimators it is well known that a good estimator is obtained by choosing weight W_j to be proportional to the reciprocal of the variance of I_j/I_{j-1}. In the present context the conditional variance is appropriate for this purpose. The conditional variance of I_j/I_{j-1}, given I_{j-1}, is σ^2/I_{j-1}, where σ^2 is the variance of the offspring distribution. This leads to the weights $W_j = I_{j-1} \sum_{i=2}^{k} I_{i-1}$. With these weights the weighted average becomes

$$\widehat{R} = \sum_{j=2}^{k} I_j \Big/ \sum_{j=1}^{k-1} I_j \,,$$

the estimator used in Section 2.7.1.

A similar conditional argument leads to a distribution-free estimate of σ^2, the variance of the offspring distribution. Conditional on $I_{j-1} = r$, the number of cases in generation j may be written $I_j = X_1 + X_2 + \cdots + X_r$, where $X_1, X_2, \dots, X_r$ are independent random variables representing the number of offspring by the r infectives of generation $j-1$. Using $\mathrm{E}(X_j) = R$ and $\mathrm{Var}(X_j) = \sigma^2$ it follows that

$$\mathrm{E}(I_j - I_{j-1}R \,|\, I_{j-1} = r) \;=\; 0 \quad \text{and} \quad \mathrm{Var}(I_j - I_{j-1}R \,|\, I_{j-1} = r) \;=\; r\sigma^2.$$

From this we deduce that

$$\widehat{\sigma}^2 \;=\; \frac{1}{k}\sum_{j=2}^{k} I_{j-1}\left(I_j/I_{j-1} - \widehat{R}\right)^2$$

is a distribution-free estimator for σ^2. For the data of Table 2.1 this gives the estimate $\widehat{\sigma}^2 = 7.65$ and standard error s.e.$(\widehat{R}) = 0.60$. The latter is similar to the standard error obtained in Section 2.7.1 under the assumption of a Geometric offspring distribution.

2.10.6 Estimating R from data on minor outbreaks

Maximum likelihood estimation of R

As in Section 2.7.2, we view the outbreak sizes in Table 2.2 as observations on independent random variables $Y_1, Y_2, Y_3, \ldots, Y_{39}$. When we assume a Poisson offspring distribution each Y_j has the Borel-Tanner distribution given by Equation (2.8), so the probability that these thirty-nine outbreak sizes are realized is

$$\Pr(Y_1 = 0) \times \Pr(Y_2 = 0) \times \cdots \times \Pr(Y_{39} = 75) \;=\; \text{constant} \times R^{199}\,\mathrm{e}^{-238R}.$$

This probability depends on R, and viewed as a function of R it is the likelihood function corresponding to the data in Table 2.2. For maximum likelihood estimation the constant in this expression has no consequence, since our interest is to determine for which value the likelihood function attains its maximum. The log-likelihood function is

$$\mathcal{L}(R) \;=\; \text{constant} + 199\ln(R) - 238R, \qquad R > 0.$$

The maximum likelihood estimate is given by the solution to the equation

$$\frac{d\mathcal{L}}{dR} \;=\; 199/R - 238 \;=\; 0,$$

giving the estimate $\widehat{R} = 199/238 = 0.836$. The large-sample theory of maximum likelihood estimation gives us the large-sample standard error

$$\text{s.e.}(\widehat{R}) \;=\; \left(-\frac{d^2\mathcal{L}}{dR^2}\right)^{-1/2}_{\{R=\widehat{R}\}} \;=\; \left(\frac{199}{\widehat{R}^2}\right)^{-1/2} \;=\; \frac{\sqrt{199}}{238} \;=\; 0.059.$$

A distribution-free standard error

Suppose we have an estimate $\hat{\theta}$ and a standard error s.e.$(\hat{\theta})$ for a parameter θ and we are interested in the parameter $\varphi = g(\theta)$. Then φ is estimated by $\widehat{\varphi} = g(\hat{\theta})$ and the Delta Method provides a large sample standard error given by

$$\text{s.e.}(\widehat{\varphi}) \;=\; \left|g'(\hat{\theta})\right| \text{s.e.}(\hat{\theta}),$$

where $\left|g'(\hat{\theta})\right|$ is the absolute value of the derivative of g evaluated at $\hat{\theta}$.

In Section 2.7.2 we used the Method of Moments to obtain the estimate $\widehat{R} = 1 - 1/\bar{y}$ of R by solving the equation $\bar{y} = 1/(1 - \widehat{R})$ for $\widehat{R}$. We can find a large sample approximation for the standard error s.e.$(\widehat{R})$ by applying the Delta Method. With $\varphi = g(\theta) = 1 - 1/\theta$ and $\hat{\theta} = \bar{y}$ the Delta Method gives

$$\text{s.e.}(\widehat{R}) \;=\; \left|g'(\bar{y})\right| \text{s.e.}(\bar{y}) \;=\; \text{s.e.}(\bar{y})/\bar{y}^2.$$

2.11 Bibliographic notes

This chapter's discussion is adapted from known results for the Galton-Watson process, a specific type of branching process. The branching process material relevant to this chapter is covered in early chapters of the republished books by Harris (2002) and Athreya and Ney (2004).

Awareness of a threshold result, akin to the Transmission Threshold Property given on page 8, goes back to Kermack and McKendrick (1927) for a deterministic epidemic model and to Bartlett (1949) for a stochastic model. Our introduction to the Transmission Threshold Property assumed that the depletion of susceptibles can be ignored when describing minor outbreaks in a large population. A derivation that avoids this assumption is given by Whittle (1955) and Becker (1977) extends his argument to a more general model.

CHAPTER 3

Minor outbreaks in a community of households

So far we have assumed that each infective has the same potential to infect others. This is not the case when the community consists of households. The primary infective of a household has more potential to infect others than a secondary infective of that household, because more susceptible household members are exposed to the primary infectives. Specifically, the primary infective in a household of size two has a chance to infect any susceptible community member outside his household *and* his household partner. If he infects his household partner then this partner has a similar chance to infect any susceptible community member of another household but he can not infect his household partner, who was infected earlier.

This difference between primary and secondary household infective suggests that one way to model transmission in a community of households is to introduce different types of infective. That is indeed a way to proceed, as we illustrate in the next chapter. In this chapter we take a simpler path, which adapts the methods and results of Chapter 2 to a community of households. The trick is to modify the allocation of new infections to infectives in a way so that every infective has the same offspring distribution.

3.1 Modified allocation of offspring

The modified allocation of offspring to infectives is explained with reference to Figure 3.1. The figure shows six households, each with two members who are susceptible before the infection is introduced. Individual A is the primary community infective. Arrows show that he infected his household partner and three members of other households. In total, he infected four individuals by direct contact. However, in this chapter we allocate offspring to an infective in a different way. We do not consider A to have four offspring. Instead, we allocate to A the three individuals he actually infected in other households *and also* all individuals subsequently infected in the households of those three individuals. We do not include the infected household partner of A as one of his offspring. In the example of Figure 3.1 this way of allocating offspring means infective A generated five offspring.

A similar allocation of offspring is used for a community with households of varying size. As above, the offspring of an infective, infective A say, include all the individuals he infects by direct contact outside his household. Each of these individuals initiates an outbreak within their own household. All other cases in those household outbreaks are also counted as offspring of infective A. However, any infected members of his own household are *not* counted as offspring of infective A, even if he was responsible for the infection.

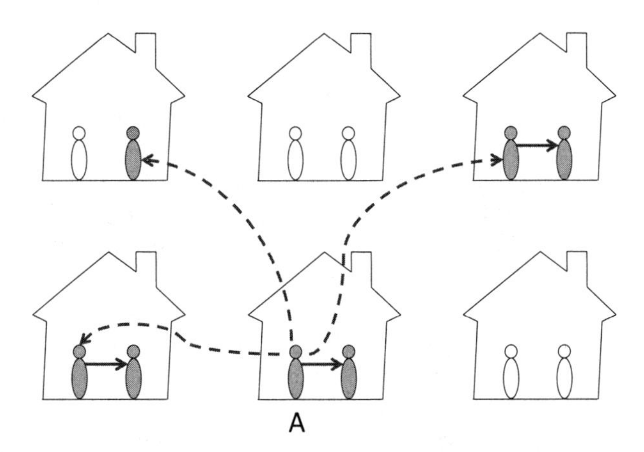

Figure 3.1 *Illustrative pattern of transmission of an infectious disease by the primary infective of a community consisting of six households. Each household contained two susceptibles prior to the introduction of the infection.*

An implicit assumption we make is that infectious contacts by an infective with community members outside his household are made at random.

3.2 Household reproduction number

With the above method of allocating offspring to infectives every infective has the same potential to generate offspring. In other words, the probability distribution for the number of offspring allocated to an infective is the same for every infective. Of course, a common offspring distribution can only be assumed in a discussion of minor outbreaks in a large community because it requires the depletion of susceptibles to be negligible.

As a consequence of having the same offspring distribution the threshold property stated on page 8 can be applied to a community of households. All we have to do is replace the reproduction number R by R_{H}, the mean number of offspring an infective is allocated by the modified allocation described in Section 3.1. We call R_{H} the *household reproduction number.*

For practical applications of this adapted transmission threshold property we need an expression for R_{H}, preferably in terms of parameters with clear demographic or epidemiological interpretations. To this end, we now express R_{H} in terms of the way susceptibles are distributed over households, the potential for transmitting the infectious disease between households and the potential for transmitting the infectious disease within households. The resulting expression provides a way to determine intervention requirements for preventing epidemics in a community of households.

Consider a community consisting of a large number of households. During the early stages of an outbreak, initiated by an external contact, each infective infects a random number of individuals in other households who then independently initiate an outbreak in their own household. This indicates that the mean of the offspring distribution is

$$R_{\text{H}} = \mu\nu_{\text{H}}, \tag{3.1}$$

where μ is the mean number of individuals an infective infects outside his household and ν_{H} is the mean outbreak size resulting in his household when a randomly selected community susceptible is infected. Equation (3.1) is formally derived in Section 3.9.1.

In Section 3.9.2 it is shown that

$$\nu_{\text{H}} = \frac{1}{n_{\text{S}}}\sum_j jH_j\nu_j, \tag{3.2}$$

where H_j is the number of households with j susceptible members, $n_{\text{S}} = \sum_j jH_j$ is the total number of susceptibles in the community and ν_j is the mean size of an outbreak in a household with j susceptible members when one of these susceptibles is infected via an external contact. Specifically, $\nu_1 = 1$ and $\nu_2 = 1 + \tilde{q}$, where $\tilde{q}$ is the probability that a primary household infective infects his susceptible household partner.

Basic household reproduction number

The distinction between basic reproduction number and effective reproduction number carries over to the household setting. In a community of households where

(i) every individual is susceptible prior to the importation of the infection,

(ii) people mix normally, and

(iii) there are no public health interventions in place,

the mean of the offspring distribution is the *basic household reproduction number*

$$R_{\text{H0}} = \mu_0\nu_{\text{H0}}.$$

The parameters μ and ν_{H} generally have smaller values than μ_0 and ν_{H0}, respectively, due to the presence of individuals with some immunity.

3.3 When are outbreaks certain to be minor?

Having derived an expression for R_{H} we are now able to rephrase the statement of the transmission threshold property given on page 8 in a form that applies to a community consisting of a large number of households.

Transmission Threshold Property for a community of households: *An outbreak arising from an imported infection is certain to be minor when* $R_{\text{H}} < 1$, *where* R_{H} *is given by (3.1) and (3.2).*

This result provides a tool for finding public health interventions able to prevent epidemics when an infectious disease is freshly introduced into a community of households. With a household setting it is necessary to consider the impact of an intervention on between-household and within-household transmission of the infection. We begin our discussion of ways to prevent epidemics by considering the fraction of individuals that must be vaccinated with a vaccine that fully protects against infection.

3.4 Mass immunization

For a community with homogeneous infectives, e.g., a community of uniformly mixing homogeneous individuals, we found that the effect mass immunization has on R is determined by v, the fraction of community members vaccinated. To quantify the effect of mass immunization on R_{H} we need to specify v, the vaccination coverage, *and* how vaccinees are distributed over the households. We illustrate this by comparing three immunization strategies in a specific setting.

3.4.1 Comparing three immunization strategies

Assume that each of the large number of households has either 0, 1 or 2 members who are susceptible to the infectious disease. Prior to an immunization campaign the effective household reproduction number for this community is $R_{\text{H}} = \mu\nu_{\text{H}}$, with

$$\nu_{\text{H}} = \frac{H_1 + 2H_2\nu_2}{H_1 + 2H_2}. \tag{3.3}$$

Note that ν_2, the mean size of an outbreak resulting in a household with two susceptibles when one of them is infected by an external contact, satisfies $1 \le \nu_2 \le 2$.

Suppose further that $H_1 = H_2$. In words, the number of households with one susceptible member equals the number of households with two susceptible members. Then the effective household reproduction number prior to an immunization campaign is

$$R_{\text{H}} = \mu(1 + 2\nu_2)/3.$$

It is proposed to have a mass immunization campaign with a vaccine that renders each vaccinee fully immune. A crucial question is: How should the limited number of vaccines be distributed over households to achieve the greatest reduction in the reproduction number? We compare three different ways of distributing vaccines, with the aims of

(i) identifying strategies that perform well and ones that do not, and

(ii) illustrating how to calculate the impact of immunization on R_{H}.

The individuals chosen for vaccination under each of the three strategies are:

`Strategy A`: All individuals belonging to a size-one household.

`Strategy B`: Both individuals in one half of the size-two households.

`Strategy C`: Exactly one individual from every size-two household.

The immunization strategies `A`, `B` and `C` reduce the reproduction number from $R_{\text{H}} = \frac{1}{3}\mu(1 + 2\nu_2)$ to

$$R^*_{\text{HA}} = \tfrac{2}{3}\mu\nu_2, \qquad R^*_{\text{HB}} = \tfrac{2}{15}\mu(3 + 2\nu_2) \quad \text{and} \quad R^*_{\text{HC}} = \tfrac{2}{3}\mu,$$

respectively. The steps in the calculation of these reproduction numbers are explained in Section 3.9.3 and shown in Table 3.1 on page 52.

Note that $R^*_{\text{HA}} = R^*_{\text{HB}} = R^*_{\text{HC}} = 2/3\mu$ when $\nu_2 = 1$. The equality of these reproduction numbers is not surprising since $\nu_2 = 1$ implies zero transmission within households and therefore the way susceptibles are distributed over households is immaterial. The common value of $2/3\mu$ for these reproduction numbers is as expected, because when within-household transmission is negligible the situation is just as in Chapter 2, and Equation (2.3) tells us that the reproduction number would be reduced to two-thirds of its pre-campaign value when one-third of all susceptibles is immunized.

The story is different when within-household transmission is possible. Figure 3.2 shows graphs of $R^*_{\text{HA}}/R_{\text{H}}$, $R^*_{\text{HB}}/R_{\text{H}}$ and $R^*_{\text{HC}}/R_{\text{H}}$ over the range $1 \leq \nu_2 \leq 2$, using the expressions given in the last row of Table 3.1, on page 52. These graphs reveal that, when $\nu_2 > 1$, the way individuals are selected for vaccination can have a substantial effect on the value achieved for the ratio of post-campaign reproduction number to its pre-campaign value.

To illustrate, note that $R^*_{\text{HA}} = 2R^*_{\text{HC}}$ for values of ν_2 near 2. This tells us how much better it is to immunize one person from every household with two susceptibles than it is to immunize the susceptible of every household with one susceptible. While this is not a surprising result in this specific setting, in more general settings such numerical comparisons form a useful basis for making infectious disease management choices.

3.4.2 Effective immunization strategies

Of the three immunization strategies compared in Figure 3.2, Strategy C is seen to provide the greatest reduction in the household reproduction

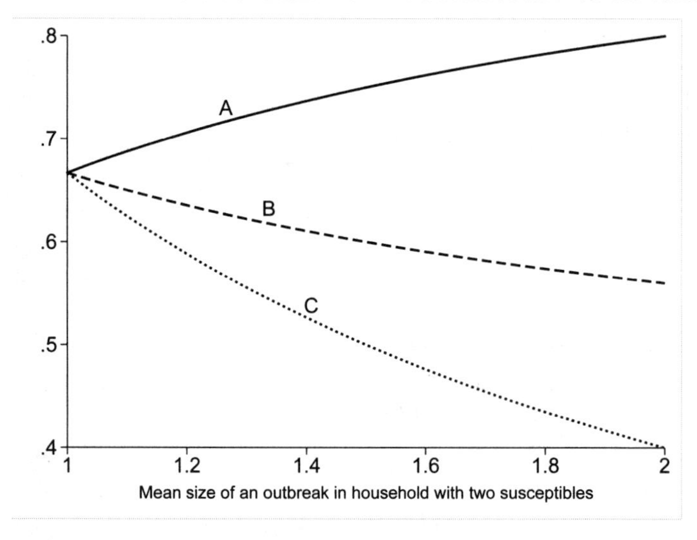

Figure 3.2 *Ratio $R^*_{\mathrm{H}}/R_{\mathrm{H}}$ for immunization strategies A, B and C as a function of ν_2, the mean size of an outbreak in a household with two susceptibles.*

number. The way individuals are selected for vaccination under Strategy C ensures that within-household transmission is minimized. This suggests that minimizing within-household transmission may be an effective way to reduce the household reproduction number in quite general settings.

Motivated by this thought, consider a setting in which the distribution of susceptibles over households is arbitrary and the reproduction number is $R_{\mathrm{H}} = \mu\nu_{\mathrm{H}}$. Any immunization campaign that immunizes a fraction v of the susceptibles reduces the mean number of individuals a primary infective infects in other households from μ to $(1-v)\mu$, irrespective of how individuals are selected for vaccination. Therefore an effective immunization campaign is one that reduces ν_{H}, the mean size of an outbreak in the household of a randomly infected community member, as much as possible.

The argument in Section 3.9.4 indicates that an effective selection of individuals is to continuously select the next susceptible for vaccination from one of the households with the largest number of remaining susceptibles at the time of the selection. From a mathematical point of view this is the best way to select individuals for vaccination. In practice this selection is difficult to implement because some households may wish to have all family members vaccinated while others do not wish anyone to be vaccinated. However, identifying this effective immunization strategy helps to point out that targeting households with a large number of susceptibles for immunization is likely to be a good way to control the infectious disease.

3.4.3 Critical vaccination coverage

We have seen that the reduction in the reproduction number achieved depends on the way individuals are selected for vaccination. It follows that the value of the critical vaccination coverage also depends on the way individuals are selected for vaccination. We illustrate this more specifically in the simple setting where all households include exactly two susceptible members. The effective household reproduction number for this community is $R_{\text{H}} = \mu\nu_{\text{H}}$, where $\nu_{\text{H}} = \nu_2$ because every household has two susceptibles.

Consider first vaccination, with a fully protective vaccine, of community members according to

`Strategy 1:` A fraction v of *households* is selected randomly and both susceptibles in every selected household are vaccinated.

This strategy reduces the reproduction number to $(1-v)R_{\text{H}}$, because μ is reduced to $(1-v)\mu$ while ν_{H} is unchanged by this form of mass immunization. The critical vaccination coverage for this strategy is the solution of $(1-v)R_{\text{H}} = 1$, namely

$$v_1^\dagger = 1 - 1/R_{\text{H}}. \tag{3.4}$$

The solid curve in Figure 3.3 shows the graph of $v_1^\dagger$ for different values of R_{H}.

Also consider vaccination, with a fully protective vaccine, according to

`Strategy 2:` A fraction v of susceptible *individuals* is selected randomly and every selected susceptible is vaccinated.

This strategy also reduces μ to $(1-v)\mu$. However, it also changes ν_{H}, because it alters the way susceptibles are distributed over households. Following vaccination according to Strategy 2 the fraction of households with 0, 1 and 2 susceptibles is given by the Binomial fractions v^2, $2v(1-v)$ and $(1-v)^2$, respectively. Substituting these fractions into Equation (3.3) we find that ν_{H} is reduced from ν_2 to $v + (1-v)\nu_2$. Therefore Strategy 2 reduces the household reproduction number to

$$(1-v)\mu[v + (1-v)\nu_2].$$

By equating this reproduction number to 1 and solving for v we obtain the critical vaccination coverage

$$v_2^\dagger = \frac{-1 + \sqrt{1 + 4(\nu_2 - 1)/\mu}}{2(\nu_2 - 1)}.$$

This critical vaccination coverage depends on the extent to which within-household transmission and between-household transmission contribute to the magnitude of R_{H}. The curves in Figure 3.3 show the graph of $v_2^\dagger$ over a range of R_{H} values when $\mu = R_{\text{H}}$ (solid curve), $\mu = \frac{3}{4}R_{\text{H}}$ (dashed curve) and $\mu = \frac{1}{2}R_{\text{H}}$ (dotted curve). The critical vaccination coverages for Strategy 1 and Strategy 2 coincide when $\mu = R_{\rm H}$, because $\nu_2 = 1$ implies that there is no within-household transmission.

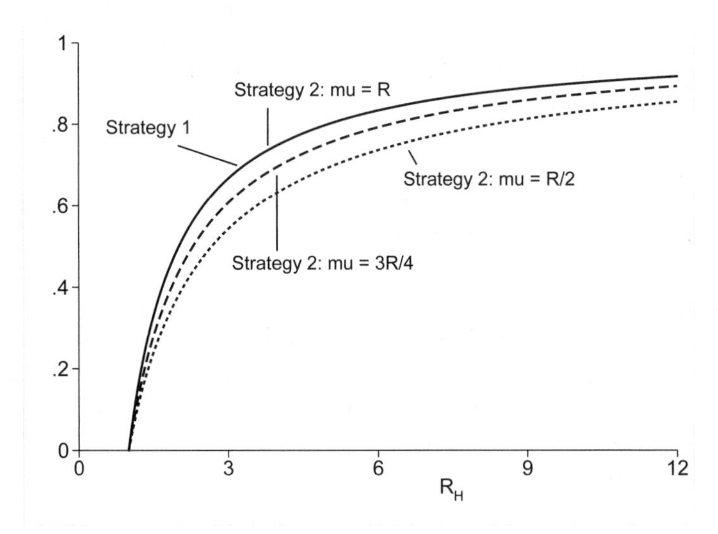

Figure 3.3 *Critical vaccination coverage for Strategy 1 and for Strategy 2, when* $\mu = R_{\rm H}$, $\frac{3}{4}R_{\rm H}$ *and* $\frac{1}{2}R_{\rm H}$. *It is assumed that all households have two susceptibles prior to the immunization campaign.*

While Strategy 2 is not the strategy with the smallest critical vaccination coverage, its critical vaccination coverage can be appreciably smaller than the critical vaccination coverage for Strategy 1. For example, suppose $R_{\rm H} = 2\frac{2}{3}$ and $\mu = \frac{1}{2}R_{\rm H} = 1\frac{1}{3}$. Then $v_1^\dagger - v_2^\dagger = \frac{5}{8} - \frac{1}{2} = \frac{1}{8}$, which means that Strategy 1 requires us to vaccinate an extra 12.5% of community members to prevent epidemics.

3.5 Are results affected by the way the infection is imported?

The transmission threshold property for the household setting, stated on page 40, requires only that we know whether, or not, the household reproduction number is currently below 1. The size of the household of which the introductory infective is a member has no impact on this property. However, the size of the introductory infective's household does have an impact on the mean of the total number of cases in a minor outbreak. It also impacts on the probability of a minor outbreak when $R_{\rm H} > 1$.

3.5.1 Mean outbreak size

Consider a community that has been free from a certain infectious disease over the recent past and $R_{\rm H}$, its household reproduction number for this disease, is less than one. Suppose one susceptible member of this community is infected by an external contact. If this primary community infective was the sole susceptible member of his household, then the expected total number of cases in this outbreak is

$$\nu = 1/(1 - R_{\text{H}}), \qquad \text{for} \quad 0 \leq R_{\text{H}} < 1,$$

by analogy with Equation (2.5).

This changes when the household of the primary infective contains other susceptibles. To illustrate, suppose his household has one other susceptible and let $\tilde{q}$ denote the probability that the primary infective infects his susceptible household partner. Then the mean of the total number of cases in the outbreak initiated by the introductory infective is

$$\nu = 1/(1 - R_{\text{H}}) + \tilde{q}/(1 - R_{\text{H}}),$$

where the first term on the right-hand side is the expected total number of cases in the transmission chain generated by the introductory infective (using the modified allocation of offspring) and the second term is the expected total number of cases in the transmission chain of the household partner.

3.5.2 Probability of a minor outbreak when $R_{\text{H}} > 1$

Consider a setting as above, but now suppose $R_{\text{H}} > 1$. By analogy with Equation (2.1) we have

$$\pi_1 = p_0 + p_1\pi_1 + p_2\pi_1^2 + p_3\pi_1^3 + \cdots \tag{3.5}$$

for π_1, the probability of a minor outbreak when the introductory infective belongs to a household with no other susceptibles. Here the offspring distribution $p_0, p_1, p_2, \ldots$ is the one obtained by allocating offspring as described in Section 3.1.

If the household of the introductory infective has one other susceptible the equation for π_2, the probability of a minor outbreak when one susceptible from a household with two susceptibles initiates the outbreak, is given by

$$\pi_2 = q\pi_1 + \tilde{q}\pi_1^2,$$

where $\tilde{q} = 1 - q$ is the probability that the primary infective infects his susceptible household partner and π_1 is determined by Equation (3.5). The first term on the right-hand side corresponds to the event that the initial infective does not infect his susceptible household partner and the second term corresponds to the event that he does infect his susceptible household partner.

3.6 Estimating R_H

The types of model we have introduced so far apply only during the early stage of an outbreak. This limits parameter estimation based on these models to data observed during the early stage of an outbreak or to observations on a collection of minor outbreaks. The method for estimating R described in Section 2.7.2 uses such data and can be adapted to provide estimates of μ and ν_H, and therefore $R_H = \mu\nu_H$.

Suppose a community has control measures in place for a certain infectious disease. These are adequate to provide periods of elimination that are interrupted only by minor outbreaks, occurring when the disease is imported by an external contact. To ensure that epidemics continue to be prevented, it is important to use such data to monitor the value of the reproduction number to check that it is maintained below 1.

Assume that data on k recent outbreaks have been collected. Each outbreak contains only a small amount of information, so we need to combine the data from all k outbreaks. Let m_j denote the number of household outbreaks with j cases, among the k observed community outbreaks.

In this notation we have a total of $m_H = \sum_j m_j$ infected households and a total of $m_C = \sum_j jm_j$ cases. These m_C cases infected a total of $m_H - k$ households. The outbreaks in the households of the k introductory infectives are excluded, because they were infected by an external contact. Therefore an estimate of μ is given by

$$\hat{\mu} = (m_H - k)/m_C.$$

The parameter ν_H is the mean size of a household outbreak and we simply estimate it by the average size of household outbreaks observed in the k community outbreaks, including the outbreaks in the households of the k introductory infectives. That is

$$\hat{\nu}_H = m_C/m_H,$$

which leads to the estimate

$$\widehat{R}_H = (m_H - k)/m_H = 1 - k/m_H. \qquad (3.6)$$

The estimate $\widehat{R}_H$ is never greater than 1, which is as expected when we are observing minor outbreaks.

3.7 Discussion

By looking at a community of households, we have in this chapter taken the first step towards showing that analogs of the transmission threshold property hold in real-world settings. The modified allocation of offspring to infectives used brings with it three nice properties for the resulting threshold parameter. Firstly, the algebraic expression for R_H has a very manageable form, which makes it well suited to ascertaining the level of public health intervention required to prevent epidemics. Secondly, this threshold parameter has a straightforward interpretation as a reproduction number, which assists in providing epidemiological insights. Finally, its interpretation as a reproduction number and its expression in terms of parameters with clear epidemiological interpretations brings with it scope for finding ways to estimate its value from available data, as shown in Section 3.6.

Our modeling has shown that a new feature arises when considering public health interventions for preventing epidemics in a community consisting of households. Some ways of selecting individuals for vaccination reduce the reproduction number effectively while other selections perform poorly. The most effective way to distribute vaccinations among individuals may not receive public acceptance, but it helps to know which allocation of vaccines to aim for when designing public health interventions. For example, we have seen that a mass immunization campaign that targets households, and vaccinates all members of selected households, usually reduces the reproduction number less than a campaign that achieves the same coverage but targets individuals. This suggests that a campaign targeting households may not be as effective as an immunization campaign that is delivered through schools or workplace.

Our illustrative examples assume small households and quite specific settings. This is done only for convenience, with the aim of making it easier to communicate new issues that arise when considering a community of households. All expressions retain an explicit form when generalized to a community with an arbitrary distribution of household size. This is an important point, because explicit formulae make the assessment of real-world control measures convenient.

To use the transmission threshold property to inform the outbreak response to a newly emerged infectious disease in a community of households, the data collected at the start of the outbreak need to be enhanced. For example, we might aim for timely reporting of daily incidences for the first 100 cases, 20 observed serial intervals, the number of different households infected, their sizes and, for 20 (say) affected households, the size of the household and the eventual number of its members infected. We also need, from demographic records, the distribution of household size in the community. Such data allow us to assess the relative role of between-household and within-household transmission, as required for the results of this chapter.

Two major reasons for including data on within-household transmission in response surveillance data are

(i) they are often a good source of observations on the serial interval, and

(ii) they inform decisions on household related interventions such as quarantining households and isolating symptomatic infectives.

3.8 Exercises

1. Consider a community with a large number of households, each of which has two susceptible members. During the early stages of an outbreak each infective independently infects 0, 1 or 2 individuals outside his household with probability 0.2, 0.3 and 0.5, respectively. A primary household infective infects the susceptible member of his household with probability 0.4.

   (a) For an individual who was infected during the early stage of an outbreak, compute

      (i) μ, the mean number of individuals he infects outside his household, and

      (ii) ν_{H}, the mean size of the outbreak in his household if he is the primary household infective.

   (b) Using the allocation of offspring to infectives described in Section 3.1, find

      (i) R_{H}, the household reproduction number, and describe circumstances under which this is a *basic* reproduction number,

      (ii) all possible values for the number of offspring that can be allocated to an infective,

      (iii) the probability distribution for the number of offspring allocated to an infective, and

      (iv) the mean of the offspring distribution found in (iii) and compare its value with the value of R_{H} computed in (i).

   (c) Compute the value of π, the probability of a minor outbreak, when the outbreak is initiated by one community member who was infected by an external contact.

   (d) Specify an immunization strategy and compute the critical vaccination coverage for your selected strategy, assuming that the vaccine is fully protective.

2. Consider a community in which, as in Section 3.4.1, households have either 0, 1 or 2 members who are susceptible to the infectious disease and the number of households with 1 susceptible equals the number with 2 susceptibles. As in Section 3.4.1, the household reproduction number is given by $R_{\text{H}} = \mu\nu_{\text{H}} = \mu(1 + 2\nu_2)/3$.
   An immunization campaign is conducted in which one-third of all individuals are selected for immunization randomly, without regard to any characteristic of their household.

   (a) Give an expression for

      (i) μ^*, the value to which μ is changed by the immunization campaign,

(ii) ν_{H}^*, the value to which ν_{H} is changed by the immunization campaign,

(iii) R_{H}^*, the value to which R_{H} is changed by this immunization campaign.

(b) Sketch the graph of $R_{\text{H}}^*/R_{\text{H}}$ against ν_2. Comment on the comparison of this graph with the graphs in Figure 3.2.

3. Two large cities, City 1 and City 2, have an immunization schedule in place to prevent measles epidemics. Minor outbreaks of measles occur from importations of the infection. Over the same two-year period these cities monitor their outbreaks of measles.

In the table below, which summarizes the data observed on the 10 outbreaks that occurred in City 1 and the 20 outbreaks that occurred in City 2, we have used m_1, m_2, m_3 and m_4 to denote the number of household outbreaks of size 1, 2, 3 and 4, respectively.

Household outbreaks of measles in two large cities over two years

City 1					City 2				
Outbreak	m_1	m_2	m_3	m_4	Outbreak	m_1	m_2	m_3	m_4
1	0	3	1	0	1	2	1	0	0
2	0	1	3	2	2	6	0	0	0
3	1	0	0	0	3	1	0	1	0
4	0	1	0	1	4	12	2	0	1
5	0	1	1	0	5	4	0	0	0
6	0	4	3	1	6	1	1	0	0
7	1	1	2	0	7	1	0	0	0
8	0	3	0	0	8	3	0	0	0
9	1	0	0	0	9	1	0	0	0
10	0	2	0	1	10	2	0	0	0
					11	2	0	0	0
					12	2	0	0	0
					13	5	1	0	0
					14	2	0	0	0
					15	0	1	1	0
					16	1	0	0	0
					17	1	0	0	0
					18	8	1	0	0
					19	2	0	0	0
					20	1	0	0	0

(a) For each city use these data to determine

(i) m_{H}, the total number of households that were infected over the two-year period, and

(ii) m_{C}, the total number of cases that were infected over the two-year period.

(b) For each city compute estimates of μ, ν_{H} and R_{H}.

(c) Interpret differences in your parameter estimates for these two cities and give plausible explanations for these differences.

4. Explain why the form of estimate $\widehat{R}_{\mathrm{H}}$ in (3.6) is not surprising when transmission of an infectious disease in a community of households is viewed as reproduction of infected households.

3.9 Supplementary material

3.9.1 Household reproduction number

Our aim is to obtain an expression for the household reproduction number based on the allocation of offspring described in Section 3.1.

Consider a newly infected individual, A say, who returns to his community which consists of a very large number of households. Let K denote the number of individuals infected by A in other households and denote the expected value $\mathrm{E}(K)$ by μ. With uniform mixing each of the offspring of A, if any, is certain to be the primary infective of their household. In the event $K = k$, where k is a positive integer, label these k primary household infectives $1, 2, \ldots, k$. Let W_j denote the size of the outbreak in the household of primary household infective j. Then the number of offspring allocated to individual A is given by

$$X = \begin{cases} 0, & \text{if } K = 0, \\ W_1 + W_2 + \cdots + W_k, & \text{if } K = k > 0, \end{cases}$$

where the W_j are independent random variables with identical probability distributions and hence the same mean, ν_{H} say. Using

$$\mathrm{E}(X \mid K = k) = \mathrm{E}(W_1 + W_2 + \cdots + W_k) = k\nu_{\mathrm{H}},$$

which also applies when $k = 0$, we find the mean number of offspring allocated to A to be

$$R_{\mathrm{H}} = \mathrm{E}(X) = \mathrm{E}[\mathrm{E}(X \mid K)] = \mathrm{E}[K\nu_{\mathrm{H}}] = \mu\nu_{\mathrm{H}}.$$

This is the household reproduction number introduced in Section 3.2; see Equation (3.1).

We now find an expression for ν_{H}.

3.9.2 The mean size of a household outbreak

Individual j, infected by primary infective A, is randomly selected from community members not in individual A's household. The size of the outbreak in the household of individual j depends on the number of susceptible members remaining in his household and the probability distribution of outbreak size in such a household. We now explore how these two chance elements contribute to the value of $\nu_{\rm H}$.

Let H_k denote the number of households with k susceptibles. The proportion of susceptibles who are members of a household with k susceptibles is $kH_k/n_{\rm S}$, where $n_{\rm S} = \sum_\ell \ell H_\ell$ is the total number of susceptibles in the community. Therefore

$$\nu_{\rm H} = \sum_k \frac{kH_k}{n_{\rm S}} \nu_k,$$

where $kH_k/n_{\rm S}$ is the probability that a randomly selected community susceptible is from a household with k susceptibles and ν_k is the mean size of a household outbreak initiated when one susceptible from such a household is infected by an external contact.

Note that $\nu_1 = 1$ and $\nu_2 = 1 + \tilde{q}$, where $\tilde{q}$ is the probability that the primary infective in a household with one other susceptible infects this household partner. Assigning values to the mean outbreak sizes $\nu_2, \nu_3, \ldots$ requires model assumptions and data. Chapter 10 gives a variety of probability models for household outbreaks.

3.9.3 Calculating the effect of three immunization strategies on $R_{\rm H}$

Each of the three immunization strategies `A`, `B` and `C` specified on page 41 immunizes one-third of the susceptible individuals in the population. This reduces the mean number of individuals an infective infects in other households from μ to $2\mu/3$. Consider now how H_1 and H_2, the number of households with 1 and 2 susceptibles, respectively, are changed by these immunization strategies. We are given that prior to the immunization campaign their values are $H_1 = H_2 = H$. After the campaign the values of H_1 and H_2 are as shown in the second row of Table 3.1. The mean household outbreak sizes $\nu_{\rm H}$, shown in row three of Table 3.1, are obtained from Equation (3.3) using these post-campaign values for H_1 and H_2. Finally, multiplying the elements in row one by the elements in row three gives the effective reproduction number for each of the three immunization strategies, as shown in row four of Table 3.1.

3.9.4 Who should be vaccinated next?

Consider a setting in which the distribution of susceptibles over households is arbitrary and the reproduction number is $R_{\rm H} = \mu\nu_{\rm H}$. Let $n_{\rm S}$ denote the total number of susceptibles in the community. We look at two scenarios for selecting one of these susceptibles for vaccination:

Table 3.1: *Effect of three immunization strategies on* R_{H}

		Strategy		
	Prior to campaign	A	B	C
Community infection	μ	$\frac{2}{3}\mu$	$\frac{2}{3}\mu$	$\frac{2}{3}\mu$
(H_1, H_2)	(H, H)	$(0, H)$	$(\frac{3H}{2}, \frac{H}{2})$	$(2H, 0)$
ν_{H}	$\frac{1}{3} + \frac{2}{3}\nu_2$	ν_2	$\frac{1}{5}(3 + 2\nu_2)$	1
Reproduction number	$R_{\mathrm{H}} = \frac{1}{3}\mu(1 + 2\nu_2)$	$R^*_{\mathrm{HA}} = \frac{2}{3}\mu\nu_2$	$R^*_{\mathrm{HB}} = \frac{2}{15}\mu(3 + 2\nu_2)$	$R^*_{\mathrm{HC}} = \frac{2}{3}\mu$
Ratio $R^*_{\mathrm{H}}/R_{\mathrm{H}}$	1	$2\nu_2/(1 + 2\nu_2)$	$(6 + 4\nu_2)/(5 + 10\nu_2)$	$2/(1 + 2\nu_2)$

Scenario $\mathcal{K}$: Vaccinate a single susceptible from one of the households with k susceptibles.

Scenario $\mathcal{L}$: Vaccinate a single susceptible from one of the households with ℓ susceptibles, where $k < \ell$.

The question is: Which scenario changes $R_{\text{H}} = \mu\nu_{\text{H}}$ the most?

Scenario $\mathcal{K}$ reduces the reproduction number to $R_{\text{H}k} = \mu_k \nu_{\text{H}k}$, while Scenario $\mathcal{L}$ reduces it to $R_{\text{H}\ell} = \mu_\ell \nu_{\text{H}\ell}$. Both scenarios reduce the total number of susceptibles to $n_{\text{S}} - 1$ and the mean number that an individual infects outside their own household is thereby reduced to $\frac{n_{\text{S}}-1}{n_{\text{S}}}\mu$. That is, $\mu_k = \mu_\ell = \frac{n_{\text{S}}-1}{n_{\text{S}}}\mu$. Any difference in the reproduction number must therefore come from a different effect on the mean size of a household outbreak.

Under Scenario $\mathcal{K}$ one of the households with k susceptibles is changed to a household with $k-1$ susceptibles. This reduces ν_{H} to

$$\nu_{\text{H}k} = \frac{1}{n_{\text{S}} - 1}[n_{\text{S}}\nu_{\text{H}} - k\nu_k + (k-1)\nu_{k-1}].$$

Similarly, for Scenario $\mathcal{L}$ we find

$$\nu_{\text{H}\ell} = \frac{1}{n_{\text{S}} - 1}[n_{\text{S}}\nu_{\text{H}} - \ell\nu_\ell + (\ell-1)\nu_{\ell-1}].$$

This gives

$$R_{\text{H}k} - R_{\text{H}\ell} = \frac{\mu}{n_{\text{S}}}[\ell\nu_\ell - k\nu_k + (k-1)\nu_{k-1} - (\ell-1)\nu_{\ell-1}]. \tag{3.7}$$

To determine which of these scenarios reduces the reproduction number the most we need to know $\nu_2, \nu_3, \ldots$. A natural way to proceed is to determine the ν_j from appropriate transmission models for household outbreaks. Some models for household outbreaks are given in Chapter 10. However, expressions for ν_j are not as simple as we would like and so, instead, we proceed here by using the approximation $\nu_j = 1 + \theta(j-1)$, with θ taking values from 0 to 1. This approximation has the desirable features of having a simple form and being able to reflect several properties of the ν_j that we know to be true.

Firstly, we know that each ν_j is close to 1 when within-household transmission is minimal, and our approximation mimics this with values of θ close to zero. Secondly, we know that each ν_j is close to j when the within-household transmission rate is high, and our approximation captures this with values of θ close to 1. Thirdly, generally we expect ν_j to increase as j increases and our approximation has that property as well. Finally, although the ν_j obtained for the household outbreak models of Chapter 10 are not generally linearly related to j, numerical exploration of the values of ν_j in such models reveals that they deviate from linearity by only a small amount.

When we substitute $\nu_j = 1 + \theta(j-1)$ into Equation (3.7) for $j = k$ and ℓ we obtain

$$R_{\mathrm{H}k} - R_{\mathrm{H}\ell} = 2\mu\theta(\ell - k)/n_{\mathrm{S}}.$$

The important observation is that this difference is never negative. This means that, if our purpose is to reduce the reproduction number as much as possible, the next susceptible to vaccinate should be a member from the household with the largest number of susceptibles. Repeated application of this result indicates that an effective immunization strategy is to continuously select each susceptible for vaccination from one of the households with the largest number of susceptibles at the time.

3.10 Bibliographic notes

Becker and Utev (1998) show that the vaccination coverage needed to prevent epidemics tends to be underestimated under the assumption of homogeneity. It is therefore important to include household structure in a model when the purpose is to estimate the critical immunity coverage in a setting where within-household transmission is substantial.

Bartoszyński (1972) introduced the idea of using a branching process to describe the transmission of an infectious disease from household to household. A related approach was used by Becker and Dietz (1995) to explore the effect of the distribution of household size on transmission and control of an infectious disease, assuming that the infectious disease is highly infectious within households. Ball et al. (1997) give a comprehensive discussion for an infectious disease with two levels of mixing, which includes a community of households as a particular case.

Becker and Starczak (1997) present a numerical way to compute optimal vaccination strategies for a community of households. A more general analysis of this problem is undertaken by Ball and Lyne (2002).

CHAPTER 4

Minor outbreaks when individuals differ

It is often necessary to allow for different types of individual in infectious disease models. For example, our model needs to keep track of elderly infectives if, as for influenza, they are known to be at greater risk of severe illness. Models also need to allow for different types of individual when there are identifiable groups who play different roles in the transmission of the infection. Such differences can have a biological source. For example, a less developed immune system in children may make them more susceptible to infection or, when infected, have a longer infectious period than infected adults. Different roles in transmission can also have a social source. For example, the frequency and types of contact schoolchildren have differs from those of adults.

Our discussion is restricted to two types of individual, because this helps to simplify the discussion. Two types are adequate to illustrate new issues that arise with different types of individual.

Types are assumed to be clearly identifiable. Examples are "young and old individuals," "males and females," "vaccinated and unvaccinated individuals" or "pregnant women and other individuals."

We begin by considering a community without a household structure.

4.1 Type-specific offspring distributions

Consider a large community that consists of two types of individual, Type 1 and Type 2. The two types of individual may differ in how susceptible they are to infection. Also, when infected, they may differ in how infectious they are to others. Type-specific differences are accommodated in a model by tailoring an offspring distribution to each type of infective. Each of these two offspring distributions need to be bivariate, because each infective can infect individuals of either type.

Let $p_1(i,j)$ denote the probability that a Type 1 infective generates a total of i offspring of Type 1 and j offspring of Type 2. Similarly, the probability that a Type 2 infective has i offspring of Type 1 and j offspring of Type 2 is denoted $p_2(i,j)$.

Associated with the two bivariate offspring distributions are four type-specific mean number of offspring. Our notation for these is as follows:

μ_{11} = mean number of Type 1 offspring produced by a Type 1 infective,
μ_{12} = mean number of Type 2 offspring produced by a Type 1 infective,
μ_{21} = mean number of Type 1 offspring produced by a Type 2 infective,
μ_{22} = mean number of Type 2 offspring produced by a Type 2 infective.

In the discussion below we find the mean matrix

$$\begin{pmatrix} \mu_{11} & \mu_{12} \\ \mu_{21} & \mu_{22} \end{pmatrix}$$

a convenient aid when specifying a model.

The means μ_{ij} are derived from the offspring distributions in the usual way. For example

$$\mu_{12} = \sum_i \sum_j j \, p_1(i,j) \, ,$$

where the summation notation indicates that the terms $j \times p_1(i,j)$ are summed over all the values of i and j for which the probability $p_1(i,j)$ is positive.

4.2 When are outbreaks certain to be minor?

The fact that we now have two bivariate offspring distributions and four type-specific means gives the impression that introducing types of individual complicates models dramatically and decreases the scope for using them to inform the control of infectious diseases. Fortunately there is good news. The most important news is, as we will see below, that a form of the transmission threshold property holds for infectious disease outbreaks when there are types of individual.

In the present setting, the probability that an outbreak initiated by a newly infected community member is minor depends on the type of the initial infective. Denote the probability of a minor outbreak by π_1 if the outbreak is initiated by a single introductory infective of Type 1, and by π_2 if the outbreak is initiated by a single introductory infective of Type 2. An argument analogous to that used in Section 2.1, for each type of introductory infective, gives the bivariate extension of Equation (2.1) to be given by the two equations

$$\pi_1 = \sum_i \sum_j p_1(i,j) \pi_1^i \pi_2^j \qquad \text{and} \qquad \pi_2 = \sum_i \sum_j p_2(i,j) \pi_1^i \pi_2^j \, . \quad (4.1)$$

These two simultaneous equations can be solved when the two bivariate distributions are specified; see Exercise 2 in Section 4.7 for an example.

An analysis of the solutions to Equation (4.1) gives the

Transmission Threshold Property when individuals come in two types: *An outbreak arising from an imported infection is certain to be minor when*

$R_{\mathrm{T}} < 1$, *where*

$$R_{\mathrm{T}} = \frac{1}{2}\left(\mu_{11} + \mu_{22} + \sqrt{(\mu_{11} - \mu_{22})^2 + 4\mu_{12}\mu_{21}}\right). \quad (4.2)$$

The form of this threshold property is similar to versions given for different settings, on pages 8 and 40. One difference is that the threshold parameter is now expressed in terms of the type-specific means μ_{11}, μ_{12}, μ_{21} and μ_{22}. Another difference is that the expression for R_{T} is less intuitive. Specifically, it does not reveal why R_{T} is a threshold parameter, nor why it is referred to as a reproduction number in the literature. We now throw some light on these questions and Section 4.8.1 explains how the form of R_{T} given by (4.2) is arrived at.

Is R_{T} a reproduction number?

As mentioned earlier, a threshold parameter need not be a reproduction number. The advantages of working with a threshold parameter that has an interpretation as a reproduction number, in some sense, are that

(i) it gives us a better chance of finding an estimator for it, and

(ii) it tends to be easier to deduce the impact that a proposed public health intervention will have on it.

To understand the sense in which the R_{T} given by (4.2) is a reproduction number consider the progress of a substantial outbreak in a community with two types of individual. For a period after the very early fluctuations in case incidence, the *fraction* of all cases in a generation that are of Type 1 tends to remain approximately the same from generation to generation. Then R_{T} is the mean number of offspring, counting both types, produced by an infective who is randomly selected from all infectives of such a generation. Section 4.8.1 elaborates on this explanation.

4.3 Mass immunization

We use vaccination, with an effective vaccine, to illustrate how this version of the transmission threshold property can be used to inform infectious disease control. Suppose a mass vaccination campaign is able to vaccinate a fraction v_1 of susceptibles of Type 1 and a fraction v_2 of susceptibles of Type 2. The effect of this campaign on the type-specific mean number of offspring is shown in Table 4.1. For example, the type-specific mean μ_{12} is changed to $(1 - v_2)\mu_{12}$. This is explained by the fact that only a fraction $1 - v_2$ of the individuals of Type 2 who were susceptible prior to the campaign are still susceptible after the campaign. Thereby the expected number of close contacts with Type 2 individuals that lead to infection is reduced by a factor of $1 - v_2$.

Mass vaccination changes the reproduction number from the pre-campaign

Table 4.1: *Type-specific mean number of offspring an infective has before and after an immunization campaign*

	Pre-campaign		*Post-campaign*	
	Type 1 offspring	Type 2 offspring	Type 1 offspring	Type 2 offspring
Type 1 infective	μ_{11}	μ_{12}	$(1-v_1)\mu_{11}$	$(1-v_2)\mu_{12}$
Type 2 infective	μ_{21}	μ_{22}	$(1-v_1)\mu_{21}$	$(1-v_2)\mu_{22}$

value R_{T}, given by Equation (4.2), to the post-campaign value

$$R_{\mathrm{T}}^* = \frac{1}{2}\left(\tilde{v}_1\mu_{11} + \tilde{v}_2\mu_{22} + \sqrt{(\tilde{v}_1\mu_{11} - \tilde{v}_2\mu_{22})^2 + 4\tilde{v}_1\tilde{v}_2\mu_{12}\mu_{21}}\right),$$

where $\tilde{v}_1 = 1 - v_1$ and $\tilde{v}_2 = 1 - v_2$. In the particular case when $v_1 = v_2$ this expression reduces to

$$R_{\mathrm{T}}^* = (1-v)R_{\mathrm{T}},$$

where v is the common value of v_1 and v_2. Equating this R_{T}^* to 1 gives the critical vaccination coverage

$$v^\dagger = 1 - 1/R_{\mathrm{T}}.$$

This form for the critical vaccination coverage is familiar from Equations (2.4) and (3.4).

The condition $v_1 = v_2$ applies when individuals are chosen for vaccination randomly, irrespectively of type. Such a selection of individuals for vaccination may be convenient in practice. However, we should be aware of the extent to which selecting individuals for vaccination in a type-specific way can reduce the critical vaccination coverage. We illustrate this with a simple model in which types differ only in susceptibility to infection. Individuals that are infected have the same potential to infect others, irrespective of their type. The source of this difference in susceptibility might be biological or a difference in hygiene, but a difference in mixing rates is unlikely to affect only susceptibility.

For convenience, it is also assumed that prior to the vaccination campaign no individuals are immune. Then the pre-campaign mean matrix may be written

$$\begin{pmatrix} \mu_{11} & \mu_{12} \\ \mu_{21} & \mu_{22} \end{pmatrix} = \begin{pmatrix} \alpha_1 f_1 & \alpha_2 f_2 \\ \alpha_1 f_1 & \alpha_2 f_2 \end{pmatrix}, \tag{4.3}$$

where f_1 denotes the fraction of community members that are of Type 1 and $f_2 = 1 - f_1$ is the fraction of Type 2 individuals. The fractions f_1 and f_2 have been included in the expression of the type-specific means to separate the "relative abundance" and "type-specific susceptibility" components of transmission. For the model with mean matrix (4.3) the expressions for

R_{T}, R^*_{T} and the overall vaccination coverage are

$$R_{\mathrm{T}} = \alpha_1 f_1 + \alpha_2 f_2, \quad R^*_{\mathrm{T}} = \tilde{v}_1 \alpha_1 f_1 + \tilde{v}_2 \alpha_2 f_2 \quad \text{and} \quad v = v_1 f_1 + v_2 f_2.$$

The smallest critical vaccination coverage is achieved by choosing the values of v_1 and v_2 so that $v = v_1 f_1 + v_2 f_2$ is minimized subject to

$$0 \leq v_1 \leq 1, \quad 0 \leq v_2 \leq 1 \qquad \text{and} \qquad R^*_{\mathrm{T}} = \tilde{v}_1 \alpha_1 f_1 + \tilde{v}_2 \alpha_2 f_2 \leq 1.$$

This minimization is a standard linear programming problem. However, we will simply use a few numerical examples to illustrate that a substantially lower critical vaccination coverage can be achieved by choosing the values of v_1 and v_2 prudently.

Assume that the reproduction number for this infectious disease in our community is $R_{\mathrm{T}} = 5$. With $v_1 = v_2 = 1 - 1/R_{\mathrm{T}} = 0.8$ the vaccination coverage is $v = v_1 f_1 + v_2 f_2 = 0.8$ and the reproduction number is reduced to $R^*_{\mathrm{T}} = 1$. When $\alpha_1 = \alpha_2$ we can not achieve $R^*_{\mathrm{T}} = 1$ with a vaccination coverage that is lower than 0.8. However, many values of f_1, α_1 and α_2 are consistent with $R_{\mathrm{T}} = 5$ and for many of these a substantially lower vaccination coverage achieves $R^*_{\mathrm{T}} = 1$. This is illustrated with five choices of parameter values in Table 4.2.

Table 4.2: *Vaccination coverage that achieves* $R^*_{\mathrm{T}} = 1$

f_1	f_2	α_1	α_2	α_2/α_1	R_{T}	v_1	v_2	R^*_{T}	$v^\dagger$
0.5	0.5	2	8	4	5	0	1	1	0.5
0.6	0.4	1.67	10	6	5	0	1	1	0.4
0.8	0.2	1.25	20	16	5	0	1	1	0.2
0.9	0.1	0.88	42.1	48	5	0	1	1	0.1
0.9	0.1	4	14	3.5	5	0.72	1	1	0.75

The first two columns of Table 4.2 show the proportion of individuals that are of Type 1 and Type 2. The values of susceptibility coefficients α_1 and α_2, shown in columns 3 three and four, are chosen to give a pre-campaign reproduction number of 5. Column five reflects the extent to which Type 2 individuals are more susceptible. In the first four examples, i.e., those given in the first four rows of the table, the reproduction number is reduced to 1 by vaccinating only Type 2 individuals. The critical vaccination coverage $v^\dagger$ is substantially smaller than 0.8 in these examples.

In the example given in the last row the fraction of individuals that are of Type 2 is small and the relative susceptibility of Type 2 individuals is lower than in the other four examples. As a consequence it is not possible to reduce the reproduction number to 1 by only vaccinating Type 2 individuals. We must also vaccinate a substantial proportion of Type 1 individuals and the resulting critical vaccination coverage of 0.75 is only marginally below 0.8.

4.4 Types of individual in a community of households

By using a modified allocation of offspring to infectives, analogous to that described in Section 3.1, we can get a relatively convenient expression for a reproduction number and a transmission threshold property for a community of households with types of individual. We illustrate this for the case with two types. Specifically, we generalize the household reproduction number $R_{\text{H}} = \mu\nu_{\text{H}}$, introduced in Chapter 3, to accommodate types of individual.

With two types of individual each of μ and ν_{H} needs to be replaced by four type-specific mean number of offspring generated. We use the following notation:

$\mu_{12} =$ mean number of Type 2 individuals a Type 1 infective generates, by direct contact, outside his household,

μ_{11}, μ_{21} and μ_{22} are defined similarly,

$\nu_{12} =$ mean number of Type 2 cases in a household outbreak initiated by the infection of a Type 1 susceptible selected randomly from the community,

ν_{11}, ν_{21} and ν_{22} are defined similarly.

With this notation the mean matrix of the type-specific allocation of offspring to infectives can be written

$$\begin{pmatrix} m_{11} & m_{12} \\ m_{21} & m_{22} \end{pmatrix} = \begin{pmatrix} \mu_{11}\nu_{11} + \mu_{12}\nu_{21} & \mu_{11}\nu_{12} + \mu_{12}\nu_{22} \\ \mu_{21}\nu_{11} + \mu_{22}\nu_{21} & \mu_{21}\nu_{21} + \mu_{22}\nu_{22} \end{pmatrix}, \tag{4.4}$$

and, by analogy with (4.2), a reproduction number is given by

$$R_{\text{HT}} = \frac{1}{2}\left(m_{11} + m_{22} + \sqrt{(m_{11} - m_{22})^2 + 4m_{12}m_{21}}\right). \tag{4.5}$$

In a manner similar to Equation (3.2) we can express the means ν_{11}, ν_{12}, ν_{21} and ν_{22} in terms of the distribution of susceptibles, of the two types, over households. We do not give the general expressions here. Exercise 3 in Section 4.7 illustrates the calculations for a specific setting.

What we have demonstrated is that it is possible to compute, using explicit expressions, a reproduction number that is also a threshold parameter for infectious disease transmission in a community of households consisting of different types of infective. Stated formally, the form of the transmission threshold property for a community of households with two types of individual is given by:

An outbreak arising from an imported infection is certain to be minor when $R_{\text{HT}} < 1$, *where* R_{HT} *is given by (4.5).*

This provides a direct way to assess the effectiveness of public health interventions without needing to resort to tedious computer simulations.

4.5 Two reproduction numbers for a community of households

Return for a moment to the setting of a community of households consisting of homogeneous individuals. In Chapter 3 we introduced the household reproduction number R_{H}, which provided us with a transmission threshold property for a community of households. We now construct a second reproduction number for this setting. The concept of "type of individual," with a suitable choice of types, is used to construct the reproduction number based on the natural allocation of offspring to an infective. That is, the offspring of an infective are taken to be those individuals who acquired their infection by a direct contact with this infective, irrespective of whether the infected individual is a household member or not.

We follow this construction with a comparison of these two reproduction numbers, with the aim of improving our understanding of the notions of reproduction number and critical vaccination coverage.

The reproduction number based on natural allocation of offspring

For convenience consider a community in which all households contain two susceptible individuals prior to the introduction of the infection. A primary household infective is defined to be a Type 1 infective and a secondary household infective is a Type 2 infective. Then the mean matrix for these two types of infective is

$$\begin{pmatrix} \mu_{11} & \mu_{12} \\ \mu_{21} & \mu_{22} \end{pmatrix} = \begin{pmatrix} \mu & \tilde{q} \\ \mu & 0 \end{pmatrix},$$

where μ is the mean number of individuals an infective infects outside his own household and $\tilde{q}$ is the probability that a primary household infective infects his household partner.

Using Equation (4.2), the reproduction number corresponding to this mean matrix is

$$R_{\mathrm{T}} = \frac{1}{2}\left(\mu + \sqrt{\mu^2 + 4\mu\tilde{q}}\right).$$

This is the reproduction number of infectives when the offspring allocated to an infective are all individuals that were infected by direct contact with this infective. The notation R_{T} is used for this reproduction number because it is a reproduction number derived for a community with two types.

Note that the concept of "type" used here is one which applies to an infective. It is not based on a general characteristic of an individual, such as male/female or young/old. The type used here is determined for an individual only when they become infected. This works here because we are using the concept of "type" merely to allow for differences in infectivity.

To illustrate how R_{T} is changed by a mass immunization campaign, suppose we conduct a campaign in which individuals are selected randomly for vaccination, with each person being selected independently with probability v. The vaccine is assumed to be fully protective. This campaign changes the mean matrix to

$$\begin{pmatrix} \mu^*_{11} & \mu^*_{12} \\ \mu^*_{21} & \mu^*_{22} \end{pmatrix} = \begin{pmatrix} \tilde{v}\mu & \tilde{v}\tilde{q} \\ \tilde{v}\mu & 0 \end{pmatrix},$$

where $\tilde{v} = 1 - v$. Using Equation (4.2) with the elements of this mean matrix gives the post-campaign reproduction number

$$R^*_{\mathrm{T}} = (1 - v)R_{\mathrm{T}}.$$

Setting $R^*_{\mathrm{T}} = 1$ gives the critical vaccination coverage

$$v^\dagger = 1 - 1/R_{\mathrm{T}}$$

for an immunization campaign that selects individuals randomly for vaccination.

Comparing immunization strategies using R_{H} and R_{T}

For the present setting the household reproduction number (3.1) is given by

$$R_{\mathrm{H}} = \mu(1 + \tilde{q}).$$

The reproduction number R_{H} differs from R_{T} because they are based on different ways of allocating offspring to an infective. We now demonstrate that both can be used to assess infectious disease control strategies, leading to similar conclusions.

Three alternative ways to progressively select individuals for vaccination are as follows:

`Strategy A`: Vaccinate both members of one of the remaining unvaccinated households.

`Strategy B`: Vaccinate an individual selected randomly from all individuals who remain unvaccinated.

`Strategy C`: Vaccinate one member of a household with two unvaccinated members. When there are no households with two susceptibles, vaccinate any one of the remaining susceptibles.

With a vaccination coverage v, the post-campaign reproduction numbers R^*_{H} and R^*_{T} take on the expressions given in Table 4.3. The calculations are explained in Section 4.8.2.

Figure 4.1 shows the curves of post-campaign reproduction numbers R^*_{H} and R^*_{T} as $v = 1 - \tilde{v}$ increases from 0 to 1, using parameter values $\mu = 2$ and $\tilde{q} = 0.8$. The graphs in pane (a) of Figure 4.1 are the curves of R^*_{H} for the three immunization strategies `A`, `B` and `C`, while the graphs in pane (b) of Figure 4.1 are the corresponding curves for R^*_{T}.

The first thing to note is that the pre-campaign reproduction numbers are $R_{\mathrm{H}} = 3.60$ and $R_{\mathrm{T}} = 2.61$, so that the curves start off at different

Table 4.3: *Post-campaign reproduction numbers for three strategies*

	R^*_{H}	$2R^*_{\mathrm{T}}$
Strategy `A`	$\tilde{v}\mu(1+\tilde{q})$	$\tilde{v}\mu+\sqrt{\tilde{v}^2\mu^2+4\tilde{v}\mu\tilde{q}}$
Strategy `B`	$\tilde{v}\mu(1+\tilde{v}\tilde{q})$	$\tilde{v}\mu+\tilde{v}\sqrt{\mu^2+4\mu\tilde{q}}$
Strategy `C`, $v\le 0.5$	$\mu[\tilde{v}+(\tilde{v}-v)\tilde{q}]$	$\tilde{v}\mu+\sqrt{\tilde{v}^2\mu^2+4\mu\tilde{q}(\tilde{v}-v)}$
Strategy `C`, $v>0.5$	$\tilde{v}\mu$	$2\tilde{v}\mu$

values for $v=0$. As the vaccination coverage v increases the reproduction numbers are reduced, at different rates, until they all meet at $v=1$ where both post-campaign reproduction numbers are zero. That's as it should be since $v=1$ implies that all community members are immune.

For each given vaccination coverage, Strategy `B` achieves a lower reproduction number than Strategy `A` and Strategy `C` achieves a lower reproduction number than Strategy `B`. This is the case for both R^*_{H} and R^*_{T}, so they both reflect a similar relative performance for the strategies. The points where the curves meet the line $R^*=1$ are of greatest interest as they give us the critical vaccination coverages for the three strategies. The critical vaccination coverage when using Strategy `A` is $v^\dagger_{\mathrm{A}}=0.72$. For strategies `B` and `C` we observe that the critical vaccination coverage is $v^\dagger_{\mathrm{B}}=0.62$ and $v^\dagger_{\mathrm{C}}=0.50$, respectively. The curves for R^*_{H} and those for R^*_{T} give exactly the same values for the critical vaccination coverage, demonstrating that we can work with either reproduction number.

There is a preference to work with household reproduction number R_{H} because calculations are easier, particularly when there are several types of individual.

4.6 Discussion

The main message to take from Chapters 2–4 is that there is a threshold property that holds for general community settings. It provides a useful tool for assessing the effectiveness of public health measures aimed at preventing epidemics. Such assessments are facilitated by the fact that

(i) a single quantity, denoted R, defines the threshold,
(ii) R has an interpretation as a reproduction number for infectives, and
(iii) R can be expressed in terms of epidemiological and demographic parameters, which lends hope to their possible estimation from data.

However, the algebraic expression for R depends on the community setting and the roles individuals of different type play in transmission.

In this chapter we introduced the transmission threshold property for a community consisting of households in which individuals may differ. Our illustrative examples are for simple settings, but analogous conclusions hold

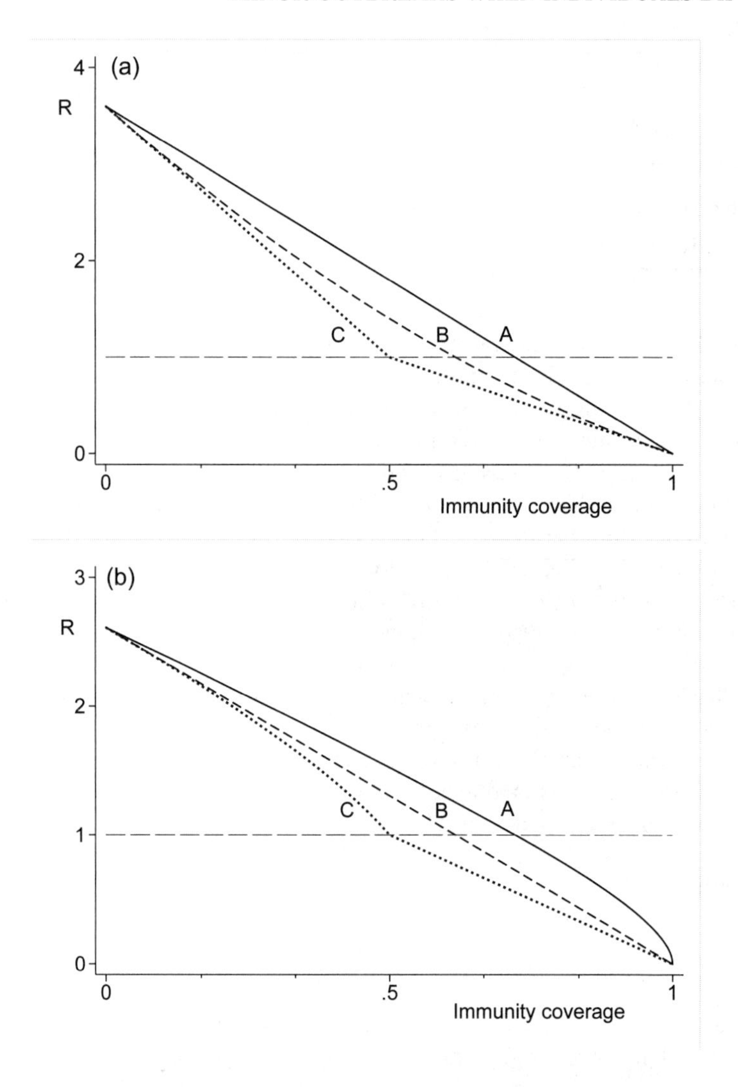

Figure 4.1 *Graphs of reproduction number* R^*_{H}, *in pane (a), and* R^*_{T}, *in pane (b), as* v, *the vaccination coverage, is increased for the three immunization strategies* `A`, `B` *and* `C` *described in the text. Parameter values are* $\mu = 2$ *and* $\tilde{q} = 0.8$.

for any number of types and any distribution of household size. Having a threshold property for a community with a network (household structure) and any number of types of individual is of considerable practical importance, because the fact that (i) this family of models is sufficient flexible to approximate any real-world community, and (ii) the threshold parameter can be computed directly means that there is unlikely to be any situation where one needs to resort to a labor-intensive, slow micro-simulation approach to guide public health measures for the prevention of epidemics.

We have seen that threshold parameters are not unique. When choosing a threshold parameter for the purpose of using it to find public health measures capable of preventing epidemics it is sensible to look for one that

(i) has a relatively simple algebraic expression, preferably in terms of standard demographic and epidemiological parameters,

(ii) has an interpretation as a reproduction number for infectives, and

(iii) can be estimated from observable data.

Data suitable for estimating a type-specific mean number of offspring, such as μ_{11}, μ_{12}, μ_{21} or μ_{22}, are often limited, because the source of an individual's infection is usually uncertain. The most fruitful way to estimate type-specific means is to express the μ_{ij} in terms of a smaller number of parameters. The next two chapters give plausible parametric forms for the μ_{ij} when types are introduced to allow for differences in susceptibility and infectivity of individuals. The need to allow for such differences arises when assessing the impact of vaccination with a partially protective vaccine and the impact of partial compliance with a public health request for social distancing. Note also that our main interest is usually not to estimate the μ_{ij}, but to estimate the initial reproduction number. Observable data are usually better suited for the estimation of R.

4.7 Exercises

1. Consider a large community with Type 1 and Type 2 individuals. Suppose the mean matrix for offspring produced by infectives of a certain infectious disease, during the early stage of an outbreak, is given by

$$\begin{pmatrix} \mu_{11} & \mu_{12} \\ \mu_{21} & \mu_{22} \end{pmatrix}.$$

The type-specific means μ_{11}, μ_{12}, μ_{21} and μ_{22} depend on demographic characteristics of the community, social characteristics of individuals and biological characteristics of the infectious disease.

(a) Describe a setting for which the mean matrix might have the form

$$(i)\ \begin{pmatrix} \mu & \mu \\ 2\mu & 2\mu \end{pmatrix} \quad (ii)\ \begin{pmatrix} \mu & 2\mu \\ \mu & 2\mu \end{pmatrix} \quad (iii)\ \begin{pmatrix} 2\mu & \mu \\ \mu & 2\mu \end{pmatrix}$$

$$(iv)\ \begin{pmatrix} \mu & 2\mu \\ 2\mu & 4\mu \end{pmatrix} \quad (v)\ \begin{pmatrix} \mu & 0 \\ 0 & 2\mu \end{pmatrix} \quad (vi)\ \begin{pmatrix} 0 & \mu \\ 2\mu & 0 \end{pmatrix}$$

(b) Give an expression for the initial reproduction number R_{T} for each of the mean-matrix scenarios in (a).

(c) Suppose a finite number of doses of a fully protective vaccine is to be used in a mass vaccination campaign with the aim of reducing the effective reproduction number.

For each of the mean-matrix scenarios in (a)

(i) propose a strategy for selecting individuals for vaccination and explain why you chose that strategy, and

(ii) determine the critical vaccination coverage for your strategy.

2. Consider a large community with two types of individual, Type 1 and Type 2. The offspring distributions, for these two types of individual during the early stage of an outbreak, are as follows:

	Offspring probability $p_1(i,j)$				Offspring probability $p_2(i,j)$		
	$j=0$	$j=1$	$j=2$		$j=0$	$j=1$	$j=2$
$i=0$	0.4	0.2	0.1	$i=0$	0.2	0.3	0.5
$i=1$	0.2	0.1	0	$i=1$	0	0	0

Find the value of

(a) the probability that a Type 1 primary infective infects at least one Type 2 individual,

(b) μ_{12}, the mean number of Type 2 individuals infected by a Type 1 infective, during the early stage of an outbreak,

(c) the initial reproduction number R_{T},

(d) π_2, the probability that an outbreak initiated by a single newly infected individual of Type 2 will be minor,

(e) π_1, the probability that an outbreak initiated by a single newly infected individual of Type 1 will be minor,

(f) the fraction of the Type 2 susceptibles that must be immunized to prevent an epidemic, if no Type 1 susceptibles are immunized.

3. In a large community 40% are Type 1 individuals and 60% are of Type 2. Everyone is susceptible to a certain infectious disease. All individuals of Type 1 live by themselves, while all Type 2 individuals live in households of size two. Type 1 individuals infect community members indiscriminately and the mean of the total number of individuals a Type 1 individual infects is 1.2. A primary Type 2 individuals infect his household partner with probability 0.8 and he also infects, indiscriminately, community members outside his household. The mean of the total number of individuals a Type 2 infective infects outside his household is 0.7.

(a) Deduce the values of μ_{11}, μ_{12}, μ_{21} and μ_{22}, the type-specific mean number of individuals an infective infects outside his household during the early stage of an outbreak.

(b) Deduce the values $\nu_{11}, \nu_{12}, \nu_{21}$ and ν_{22}, the type-specific mean number of cases in a household outbreak.

(c) Compute the household reproduction number R_{HT}.

(d) Suppose a mass immunization campaign, with a vaccine that is fully protective against this infectious disease, is conducted and achieves a coverage of v. Compute the critical vaccination coverage when

(i) only Type 1 individuals are vaccinated,

(ii) both members of a selection of households of size two are vaccinated.

4. Equation (4.2) gives the reproduction number for a community with types of individual as

$$R_{\text{T}} = \frac{1}{2}\left(\mu_{11} + \mu_{22} + \sqrt{(\mu_{11} - \mu_{22})^2 + 4\mu_{12}\mu_{21}}\right).$$

Suppose that Type 1 and Type 2 infectives infect the same mean number of Type 1 individuals, i.e., $\mu_{11} = \mu_{21} = \mu_1$, and also infect the same number of Type 2 individuals, i.e., $\mu_{12} = \mu_{22} = \mu_2$.

(a) Simplify the expression for R_{T} for this situation.

(b) Verify that the transmission threshold property reduces to that for homogeneous individuals.

Explain why you would expect this result.

5. A large community consists of households, each with two individuals that are susceptible to a certain infectious disease. The rate of within-household transmission differs among households. The probability that a primary household infective infects his household partner is $\tilde{q}_1$ in 70% of the households, the Type 1 households, and $\tilde{q}_2$ in all other households, the Type 2 households. Every infective infects a mean of μ individuals outside his household.

(a) Find an expression for the household reproduction number for the infectious disease in this community.

(b) Suppose $\mu = 0.96$, $\tilde{q}_1 = 0.2$ and $\tilde{q}_2 = 0.9$ and an immunization campaign, with a fully protective vaccine, is to be conducted.

(i) Describe how individuals should be chosen for vaccination so that the post-campaign reproduction number is reduced to 1 with the smallest vaccination coverage.

(ii) Compute the critical vaccination coverage for this optimal vaccination strategy.

4.8 Supplementary material

4.8.1 A multitype transmission threshold

A bivariate extension of the approach used in Section 2.10.1 can determine when Equations (4.1) imply that $\pi_1 = \pi_2 = 1$. This technical analysis is not given here. Instead, we simply adapt a well-known result from branching processes to deduce a multitype threshold property for infectious disease transmission.

Recall that population growth of infectives in a large community, during the early stage of an outbreak, is well approximated by a branching process. A branching process can become extinct after a finite number of births. In the context of infectious diseases this "extinction" of the population of infectives is taken to be a "minor outbreak."

It is well known that a multitype branching process becomes extinct with certainty when the largest eigenvalue of the mean matrix is less than one. Translating this to the infectious disease context of this chapter, where we have two types of individual, it means that an outbreak will be minor if the largest eigenvalue of the mean matrix

$$\begin{pmatrix} \mu_{11} & \mu_{12} \\ \mu_{21} & \mu_{22} \end{pmatrix}$$

is less than one. The two eigenvalues of this mean matrix are given by the solutions to the quadratic equation

$$x^2 - (\mu_{11} + \mu_{22})x + \mu_{11}\mu_{22} - \mu_{12}\mu_{21} \; = \; 0. \tag{4.6}$$

Its largest solution is the quantity R_{T} given by Equation (4.2), which is therefore the threshold parameter.

In what sense is R_{T} a reproduction number?

For a branching process that grows without limit, it is known that the proportion of individuals of each type converges to a fixed value. This steady distribution of types is often approximately true after only a few generations. Consider a generation G in this phase of the outbreak and let the number of Type 1 and Type 2 individuals in generation G be n_1 and n_2. The expected total number of offspring generated by these $n_1 + n_2$ infectives is

$$n_1(\mu_{11} + \mu_{12}) + n_2(\mu_{21} + \mu_{22}) \; = \; (n_1 + n_2)R, \tag{4.7}$$

where we have introduced a quantity R to represent the mean number of offspring per infective. That is, R can be interpreted as a reproduction number, averaged over the two types of infective.

To preserve the fraction of Type 1 infectives as we go from generation G to the next generation we need the fraction of the Type 1 infectives in the next generation to be $n_1/(n_1+n_2)$. This gives the equation

$$n_1\mu_{11} + n_2\mu_{21} = n_1 R. \tag{4.8}$$

By dividing all terms in Equations (4.7) and (4.8) by n_1 we obtain two equations that depend on the two variables R and n_2/n_1. Eliminating n_2/n_1 and simplifying the resulting equation leads to

$$R^2 - (\mu_{11} + \mu_{22})R + \mu_{11}\mu_{22} - \mu_{12}\mu_{21} = 0.$$

This is the same as Equation (4.6), the equation for the threshold parameter R_{T}. Therefore, it is in the sense of R, as indicated by (4.7), that R_{T} is a reproduction number.

In summary, R_{T} may be thought of as the mean number of offspring produced by an individual who is randomly selected from all infectives of a generation falling into the phase of the epidemic where the number of infectives has just started to build up.

4.8.2 Post-campaign reproduction numbers of Table 4.3

Consider a community consisting of households of size two with all members susceptible when a fraction v of individuals is vaccinated according to the selection Strategy A, B or C, defined on page 62. Our task is to derive the expressions for the post-campaign reproduction numbers R_{H}^* and R_{T}^* given in Table 4.3, on page 63, assuming the vaccine is fully protective against infection.

Household reproduction number R_{H}

The pre-campaign expression for the household reproduction number R_{H} is $\mu\nu_{\mathrm{H}}$. With a vaccination coverage v, each of the immunization strategies A, B and C reduces μ to $\tilde{v}\mu$. The effect on the mean size of the household outbreak depends on the particular immunization strategy adopted.

Following vaccination according to Strategy A each primary infective has a susceptible in his household and the mean size of the household outbreak is $1+\tilde{q}$, where $\tilde{q}$ is the probability that the primary infective infects his household partner. Therefore $R_{\mathrm{H}}^* = \tilde{v}\mu(1+\tilde{q})$.

Following vaccination according to Strategy B the post-campaign fraction of households with 0, 1 and 2 susceptibles is the Binomial fraction v^2, $2v\tilde{v}$ and $\tilde{v}^2$, respectively. Therefore the probability that a primary infective has a susceptible household partner is $2\tilde{v}^2/(2\tilde{v}^2+2v\tilde{v}) = \tilde{v}$ and $R_{\mathrm{H}}^* = \tilde{v}\mu(1+\tilde{v}\tilde{q})$.

Following vaccination according to Strategy C a primary household infective has no susceptible household partner when $v > 0.5$, so that each household outbreak is of size one and $R_{\mathrm{H}}^* = \tilde{v}\mu$. When $v \leq 0.5$ the post-campaign fraction of households with 1 and 2 susceptibles is $2v$ and $1-2v$, respectively. Therefore when a randomly selected susceptible is infected that person has a susceptible household partner with probability $2(1-2v)/[2v+2(1-2v)] = 1-v/\tilde{v}$. This gives a post-campaign household reproduction number of $R^*_{\mathrm{H}} = \tilde{v}\mu[v/\tilde{v}+(1-v/\tilde{v})(1+\tilde{q})] = \mu[\tilde{v}+(\tilde{v}-v)\tilde{q}]$.

Infectious-contact reproduction number R_{T}

The pre-campaign expression for the reproduction number R_{T} is obtained by substituting the elements of mean matrix

$$\begin{pmatrix} \mu_{11} & \mu_{12} \\ \mu_{21} & \mu_{22} \end{pmatrix} = \begin{pmatrix} \mu & \tilde{q} \\ \mu & 0 \end{pmatrix}$$

into Equation (4.2).

To specify the post-campaign expressions for this reproduction number we need to deduce how vaccination alters each of the elements of the above mean matrix and substitute these modified type-specific mean number of offspring into Equation (4.2).

Observe that a campaign with vaccination coverage v has the effect of changing μ to $\tilde{v}\mu$, irrespective of how susceptibles are selected for immunization. We deduce that each of the immunization strategies changes μ_{11} and μ_{21} to $\tilde{v}\mu$, while μ_{22} remains 0.

The effect of vaccination on the type-specific mean μ_{12} depends on the particular immunization strategy adopted.

Following vaccination according to Strategy A households have either 0 or 2 susceptibles, so any individual infected will have a susceptible household partner. Therefore μ_{12} remains $\tilde{q}$ for Strategy A.

Under Strategy B the number of households with 0, 1 and 2 susceptibles is $\tilde{v}^2$, $2\tilde{v}v$ and v^2, respectively. Therefore, the fraction of susceptibles with a susceptible household partner is $2\tilde{v}^2/[2\tilde{v}v+2\tilde{v}^2) = \tilde{v}$. This causes μ_{12} to change to $\tilde{v}\tilde{q}$.

Finally, consider immunization according to Strategy C, with a fraction v of individuals vaccinated. When $v > 0.5$ Strategy C leaves no households with two susceptibles and μ_{12} becomes 0. On the other hand, when $v \leq 0.5$ a fraction $2v$ of households has one member immunized. Therefore, the fraction of all remaining susceptibles who have a susceptible household partner is $2(1-2v)/[2v+2(1-2v)] = 1-v/\tilde{v}$, from which we deduce that μ_{12} changes to $(1-v/\tilde{v})\tilde{q}$.

Substituting the post-campaign expressions for μ_{11}, μ_{12}, μ_{21} and μ_{22} into Equation (4.2) gives the expressions for R^*_{T} shown in Table 4.3.

4.9 Bibliographic notes

Generalizations of the results to several types of individual and to an arbitrary distribution of household size are given in Becker and Hall (1996) and Hall and Becker (1996). Parameter estimation for these models is considered by Britton and Becker (2000).

CHAPTER 5

Transmission intensity function

We now take the first step towards describing the dynamics of disease transmission over calendar time and ways to assess the impact of time-dependent public health responses. Specifically, we introduce a function that, roughly speaking, describes how the chance that a particular infective infects a given susceptible changes over time. We call this function the *transmission intensity function.* The form of this function depends on the type and frequency of social interaction between these two individuals, the progress of pathogen shedding by the host and the ease with which pathogen ingested by the susceptible is able to develop within him. The infectiousness of an infective changes over time because the rate at which he sheds pathogen varies over time. Social interaction between the two individuals may also change over time. For example, they may have fewer close contacts while the infective is symptomatic.

5.1 Describing transmission intensity by a function

To introduce the notion of transmission intensity function we consider two specific community members, infective A and susceptible B. Susceptible B is at risk of being infected by A. Over the duration of A's infectious period, the chance of B being infected from another source is assumed negligible compared to the chance of being infected by A.

Let u denote the time since A was infected. Given that B is still susceptible at time u, the chance that A transmits the infection to B during the small time increment $(u, u + \delta)$ is approximated by

$$\Pr(\text{A infects B}) \;=\; \psi(u)\,\delta \;=\; 1 - \Pr(\text{A does not infect B}), \qquad (5.1)$$

with the approximation improving as the positive incremental time duration δ becomes smaller. The function $\psi(u)$ reflects how the chance that A infects B depends on the post-infection time u. Expressed another way, the function $\psi(u)$ describes the time-dependent transmission intensity between this infective-susceptible pair.

We call $\psi(u)$ a *transmission intensity function.* It is sometimes useful to think of it as a measure of the transmission intensity infective A *exerts* on B, or the transmission intensity B is *exposed* to from infective A.

Note that $\psi(u)$ may differ for different infective-susceptible pairs. We need more than one function to describe the intensity of transmission between infective-susceptible pairs when individuals are of different type. We also need more than one transmission intensity function when two individuals may be in the same household or different households.

Typically, the transmission intensity function is zero at the time when A is infected and remains zero while the pathogen establishes itself within host A. The time immediately following infection, while the newly infected host sheds no pathogen, is the latent period. The latent period ends and the *infectious period* begins when shedding begins. The transmission intensity function marks this transition by becoming positive, and then typically increases to a peak, where it may remain for a while before declining. The transmission intensity returns to zero when the infectious period ends, but would become zero earlier if the infective is isolated prior to the end of his infectious period.

A transmission intensity acting between infective A and B is zero when B is immune.

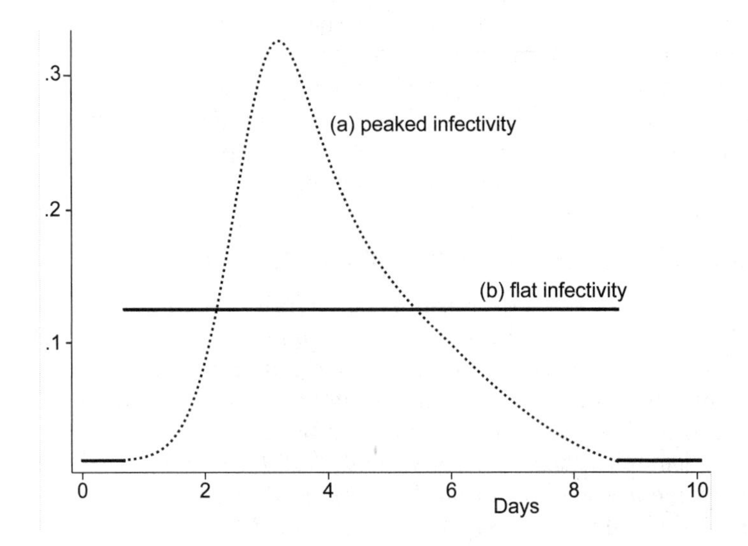

Figure 5.1 *Two transmission intensity functions with the same latent and infectious periods. In (a) infectivity changes over the infectious period. In (b) infectivity is constant over the infectious period.*

Figure 5.1 shows two transmission intensity functions. Both functions indicate a short latent period of 0.7 days, followed by an infectious period of eight days. The dotted transmission intensity curve increases from zero to a peak and then declines back to zero, in the way we might expect pathogen shedding by the host to rise and then decline as the host's immune system responds. This explanation indicates that change in the transmission intensity over time is often driven largely by the changing illness of the infective. The solid curve indicates a constant infectivity for the duration of the infectious period. Flat infectivity is often assumed in infectious disease models, because it is simple and the true pattern of infectiousness is often unknown.

For some diseases the infectiousness over time has a different pattern. For example, observations on HIV RNA copies per milliliter of plasma suggest that, in the absence of intervention, transmission intensity functions of human immunodeficiency virus (HIV) are bimodal. This means the function has two peaks. In the first few weeks after an HIV infection infectiousness is thought to follow a pattern similar to the dotted curve in Figure 5.1. During this time patients may report influenza-like symptoms. Instead of declining to zero from its peak, infectiousness settles at a lower positive value for some years before rising again as the host's immune system becomes feeble.

5.2 Estimating the transmission intensity function

It is very useful to know how the transmission intensity between infective-susceptible pairs changes over time when considering strategies to control an infectious disease, as we will see. We are therefore interested in estimating the shape of the transmission intensity function from data.

Estimating the transmission intensity function from observed incidence data is hampered by the fact that this is a function of "time since infection" and the time of infection is usually not observed. The time reported in incidence surveillance may be (i) the time of symptom onset, (ii) the time when the case presented or (iii) the time when the laboratory conducted the diagnostic test. These are often only approximate indicators of the time of infection. As a consequence, to estimate the transmission intensity function from available data we usually need to make some assumptions, using current knowledge of the disease characteristics to guide us. We illustrate this by estimating the transmission intensity function for measles from data on pairs of children in households.

The data used here were collected by Hope Simpson in the Cirencester area over the period 1946–52 and presented by Bailey (1975). They relate to outbreaks in 264 households containing two children under the age of fifteen. There were 45 households with a single case and the time duration, in days, between cases for 187 households with two cases are shown in Figure 5.2. Thirty-two households with two cases whose symptoms appeared within 5 days of each other have been excluded, based on the assumption that cases in such outbreaks were infected simultaneously by an external source and therefore data from these outbreaks are not informative about the transmission intensity between household pairs.

The data in Figure 5.2 are actually observed frequencies of the *serial interval*, which is the duration of time between onset of clinical symptoms in the primary case and symptom onset in the secondary case. We assume

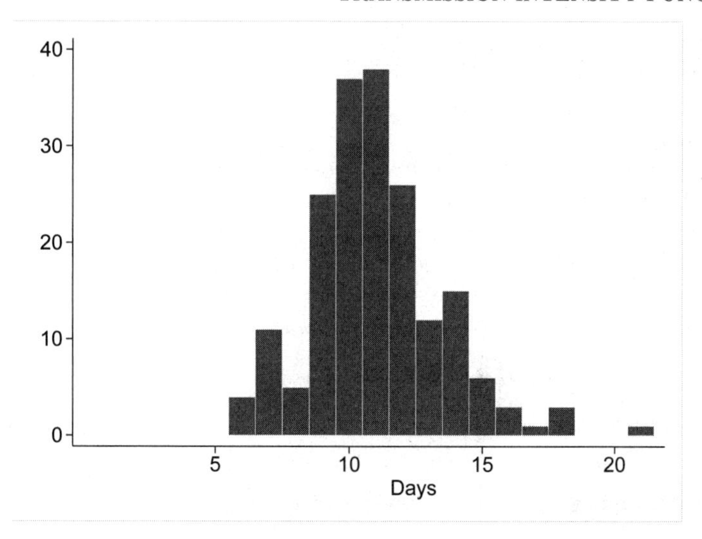

Figure 5.2 *Frequency counts for the duration of time between the detection of measles cases in households of size two.*

that the serial interval is a good reflection of the interval between the time of infection of the primary household case and the time of transmission to the secondary case. Specifically, we take "days" on the horizontal axis of Figure 5.2 to be the number of days between infection of the two household cases.

We assume that the chance of infection of the household partner from an external source is negligible when compared with the chance of infection from the primary household case. We also assume that the transmission intensity between pairs is the same in each household.

The data in Figure 5.2 are daily frequencies. It is therefore natural to assume a piecewise-constant form for the transmission intensity function. That is, we assume that the transmission intensity function $\psi(u)$ takes the value ψ_j on day j. By assumption $\psi_0 = \psi_1 = \cdots = \psi_5 = 0$, while the parameters $\psi_6, \psi_7, \ldots$ need to be estimated from the data. The values of the estimates $\widehat{\psi_6}, \widehat{\psi_7}, \ldots, \widehat{\psi_{21}}$, obtained by the method described in Section 5.6.1, are displayed by the estimated piecewise-constant transmission intensity function shown in Figure 5.3.

There is no biological or social basis for the daily rises and falls on successive days in the estimated piecewise-constant transmission intensity function. These fluctuations are likely to be due to chance. It is therefore sensible to smooth the estimates. We do so here by running a moving average over the estimates. Set $\hat{\psi}_5 = \widehat{\psi_{22}} = 0$ and define smoothed estimates of

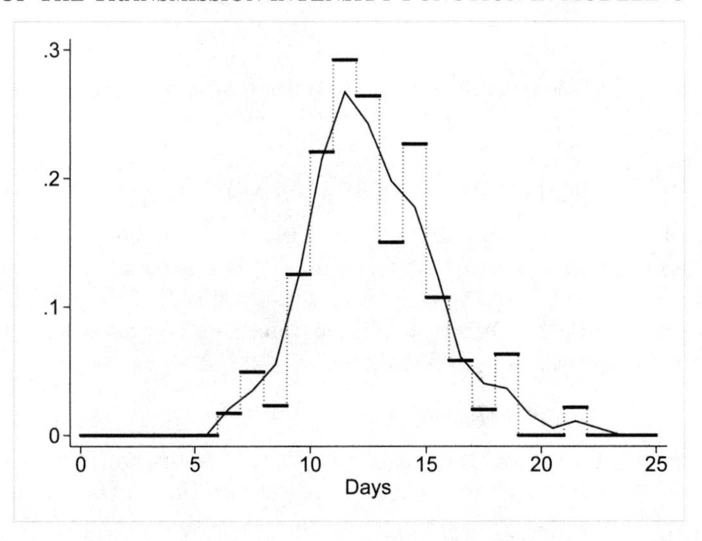

Figure 5.3 *Estimated piecewise-constant transmission intensity functions and a smoothed version of it.*

$\psi_6, \psi_7, \ldots, \psi_{21}$ by the moving weighted averages

$$\overline{\psi}_j = 0.25\widehat{\psi}_{j-1} + 0.5\widehat{\psi}_j + 0.25\widehat{\psi}_{j+1}, \qquad \text{for } j = 6, 7, \ldots, 21. \tag{5.2}$$

The $\overline{\psi}_j$ values are shown in Table 5.2, on page 86, and the continuous solid curve in Figure 5.3 is a plot of these values joined by linear segments. The resulting curve is a more plausible pattern of infectiousness over time since infection.

5.3 Role of the transmission intensity function in modeling

5.3.1 Probability of avoiding infection by a given infective

We defined the "transmission intensity function" with reference to a pair of individuals, A and B, where A is the infective. We now consider how the transmission intensity function enters a description of the probability that susceptible B avoids being infected by A over a specified time interval. For this discussion we assume that the chance of B being infected from another source during A's infectious period is negligible, merely to simplify the explanation.

From Equation (5.1) we deduce that the probability of B not having an infectious contact with A in the small time increment $(u, u+\delta)$ is approximately $1-\psi(u)\,\delta$. In Section 5.6.2 we use this probability for each of many time increments that make up the interval from $u=0$ to $u=t$ to deduce that

$$q(t) = \Pr(\text{B is not infected by A by time } t) = \exp\big[-\Psi(t)\big], \tag{5.3}$$

where

$$\Psi(t) \;=\; \text{area under the graph of } \psi(u) \text{ between } u = 0 \text{ and } u = t.$$

We call $\Psi(t)$ the *cumulative transmission intensity function.* It is a measure of the total amount of transmission intensity B has been exposed to from A over the interval from the time A was infected until t time units later.

The probability that infective A has an infectious contact with individual B before A's infectious period ends is

$$\tilde{q} = 1 - \exp(-\Psi), \tag{5.4}$$

where Ψ = total area under the graph of $\psi(u)$. Note the abbreviated notation. The area $\Psi(u_{\text{L}} + u_{\text{I}})$, where u_{L} is the duration of the latent period and u_{I} is the duration of the infectious period, is simply written Ψ.

The expressions for $q(t)$ and $\tilde{q}$ suggest that the area under the transmission intensity function plays a key role in describing the extent to which an infectious disease is transmitted through a household or a large community. This is confirmed by results that follow.

We introduced the concept of transmission intensity function in terms of a specific infective-susceptible pair of individuals. To describe the progress of the spread of an infectious disease through a community over calendar time we need to think in terms of the collection of all transmission intensities acting between infective-susceptible pairs at each point in time. The next two sections look at notions of aggregated transmission intensity, and their role in describing the initial progress of an outbreak.

5.3.2 *The aggregated transmission intensity a primary infective exerts*

Consider a uniformly mixing community consisting of n homogeneous susceptibles and one newly infected primary infective A, where n is large. We look at the potential this primary infective has to infect susceptibles of the community.

Let B be any *specific* susceptible community member. For this setting it makes sense to have the transmission intensity between A and B decrease as n increases. To reflect this dependence on n we modify the form of Equation (5.1) to

$$\Pr(\text{A infects B}) \;=\; \frac{1}{n}\psi_{\Sigma}(u)\,\delta \;=\; 1 - \Pr(\text{A does not infect B}). \tag{5.5}$$

Our assumption of a uniformly mixing community of homogeneous individuals implies that the transmission intensity A exerts on each community susceptible is the same, and described by $\frac{1}{n}\psi_{\Sigma}(u)$.

Equation (5.5) acknowledges that when n is large there is only a very small chance that A has a contact with the specific individual B in the time increment $(u, u+\delta)$, because A shares his contacts randomly and equally among all community members. By summing over all community susceptibles we find that the chance of A having an infectious contact with one of the susceptibles during the short time increment $(u, u+\delta)$ is approximately

$$\Pr(\text{A infects 1 person}) \;=\; \psi_{\Sigma}(u)\,\delta \;=\; 1-\Pr(\text{A infects no one}), \qquad (5.6)$$

with the approximation improving as δ becomes smaller. The chance that primary infective A infects more than one individual in this short time increment is negligible, when compared with $\psi_{\Sigma}(u)\,\delta$.

It is important to emphasize that $\psi_{\Sigma}(u)$ does not describe the transmission intensity between an infective-susceptible pair. Rather, it describes the *aggregated transmission intensity* that primary infective A exerts on all community susceptibles, collectively. The subscript Σ is there to remind us that $\psi_{\Sigma}(u)$ is obtained by summing n transmission intensities between pairs.

With the chance of a transmission given by (5.6), the mean number of individuals infected by primary infective A in the time increment $(u, u+\delta)$ is approximately

$$0 \times [1-\psi_{\Sigma}(u)\,\delta] + 1 \times \psi_{\Sigma}(u)\,\delta \;=\; \psi_{\Sigma}(u)\,\delta.$$

The number of individuals infected by the primary case over the duration of his infectious period is obtained by summing the mean number infected in each of a large collection of non-overlapping time increments that cover the infectious period; see Section 5.6.3. It follows that the primary infective has a mean number of offspring given by

$$\Psi_{\Sigma} \;=\; \text{total area under the graph of } \psi_{\Sigma}(u),$$

approximately. The word “approximately” is added because, strictly speaking, the aggregated transmission intensity A exerts starts to decline as primary infective A infects community members. However, this decline is negligible when n is large and A infects only a few individuals.

Note that, in this setting, $\Psi_{\Sigma} = R_0$ when no public health interventions are in place, because we assumed that all other individuals are susceptible.

Again, it is the area under the graph of a transmission intensity function that comes into play.

5.3.3 Within and between household transmission

We need more than one functional form to describe the transmission intensity between infective-susceptible pairs when the community has structure or types of individual. This is now illustrated for a simple setting.

Consider the transmission of an infectious disease amongst homogeneous individuals of a community partitioned into households. For convenience, assume every household is of size two and all individuals are susceptible when one community susceptible is infected by an outside contact.

We allocate to each primary household infective *two* transmission intensity functions expressed by $\mu\,\omega(u)$ and $\beta_{\text{H}}\omega(u)$, where the function $\omega(u)$ is non-negative and standardized so that the total area under its graph is one. The requirements on $\omega(u)$ are imposed so that intensities $\mu\,\omega(u)$ and $\beta_{\text{H}}\omega(u)$ are uniquely defined and $\omega(u)$ has a useful interpretation.

The function $\mu\,\omega(u)$ describes the transmission intensity between this primary household infective and, collectively, all individuals outside his household. That is, $\mu\omega(u)$ is similar to the aggregated transmission intensity function $\psi_{\Sigma}(u)$ introduced in Section 5.3.2.

The function $\beta_{\text{H}}\,\omega(u)$ describes the transmission intensity between this primary household infective and his household partner. That is, $\beta_{\text{H}}\,\omega(u)$ is similar to $\psi(u)$, the function introduced in Section 5.3.1 to describe the transmission intensity between a specific infective and a specific susceptible.

If the primary household infective infects his household partner, the latter also exerts an aggregated transmission intensity $\mu\,\omega(u)$ on the collection of individuals outside his household. The transmission intensity exerted by the infected household partner within his household is zero, because in the setting considered here there are no susceptibles remaining in the household.

The function $\omega(u)$ is called the *infectivity profile.* It captures the pattern of the level of infectiousness of an infective over time. The shape of the infectivity profile is determined primarily by changes in the shedding of pathogen over time and any change in mixing rate of the host due to feeling unwell or being overtly symptomatic.

The parameters β_{H} and μ are static parameters, determined by biological and social components of transmission. In terms of social interaction, β_{H} depends on the rate at which the primary infective and his household partner have close contacts, while μ depends on the rate at which the infective has close contacts with members of the community outside his household. The dependence of β_{H} and μ on biological factors are determined by characteristics of the infectious disease.

The total area under the graph of $\mu\omega(u)$ is μ, the mean number of new infections the primary infective generates outside his household over his entire infectious period. This interpretation of μ applies to the early stage of an outbreak, because the mean number infected needs to be adjusted for the depletion of susceptibles during the later stage of large outbreak. From Equation (5.4) we see that the probability of the primary case infecting his household partner is $\tilde{q} = 1 - \exp(-\beta_{\text{H}})$. In the present notation, the household reproduction number for this community is

$$R_{H0} = \mu[2 - \exp(-\beta_H)].$$

It is the basic household reproduction number because we assumed that, apart from the primary infective, all individuals are initially susceptible.

By way of summary, we have shown that R_H, a key parameter of transmission, can be expressed in terms of characteristics of the two transmission intensities. Again, it is the area under the graph of the transmission intensity functions that plays a key role in this relationship.

5.4 Discussion

This chapter introduces two related concepts, the transmission intensity function and the infectivity profile. These functions provide the natural vehicle for incorporating the effect of public health interventions into an infectious disease model. They are particularly useful when considering time-dependent public health interventions such as isolating infectives upon show of symptoms or quarantining a household when its first case is detected. Chapters 6 and 7 contain several demonstrations of how these functions help us when assessing the impact of such public health interventions.

It is important to appreciate that the transmission intensity function introduced in this chapter has biological and social-mixing components. Specifically, the function describing the transmission intensity between an infective A and a susceptible B depends on

(i) the rate at which A and B have close contact,
(ii) the rate at which A sheds pathogen, and
(iii) the chance that pathogen is transferred to B during a close contact and subsequently able to multiply within B.

We need to be aware of these associations when setting up a model. For example, the dependence on (i) indicates that the transmission intensity between infective A and susceptible B depends on their type and whether they share a household or not. We must also be aware of these associations when interpreting the transmission intensity function. For example, the rapid decline following peak infectiousness in the dotted curve of Figure 5.1 may be due to a combination of

(i) reduced shedding of pathogen following an immune response, and
(ii) reduced social mixing triggered by onset of symptoms.

Sections 5.2 and 5.6.1 describe a way to estimate a transmission intensity function without restricting the shape of the function. This approach has appeal because it does not preclude functions with an unexpected shape. A disadvantage is that it relies on having a substantial amount of data of a specific kind. An alternative approach is to restrict attention to a family of parametric models for the transmission intensity function. This has the advantage of requiring only a small number of parameters to be estimated.

A parametric approach often provides more precise estimates, provided the adopted family of models includes shapes that are close to the shape of the true transmission intensity function.

One way to protect against a poor choice when selecting a family of transmission intensity functions is to use the underlying biology that drives the changing infectivity to guide the model choice. Models formulated with reference to the mechanism that generates the data have the added attraction that their parameters have biologically meaningful interpretations and the impact of proposed public health interventions can often be reflected more naturally in such models. It may also provide the opportunity to make use of other sources of data for the purpose of estimating model parameters. Exercise 8 in Section 5.5 illustrates one way to use the underlying biology to formulate a form for the infectivity profile. It uses the population dynamics of the pathogen within the host.

The transmission intensity function allows us to describe the progress of transmission over calendar time. Exercise 9 in Section 5.5 illustrates this by deriving the probability distribution of the outbreak size in a small household at calendar time t. This allows us to quantify the progress of the outbreak, either in terms of the changing probability distribution for the number infected or, by way of summary, in terms of the mean size of the outbreak over time. What emerges is that a stochastic description of the progress of an outbreak is complicated, even for an outbreak evolving independently within a household of size three. This complexity increases dramatically as the community size increases. In Chapter 8 we sidestep this difficulty by using simplified models that are manageable, but contain the features that are essential for assessing infectious disease control measures.

5.5 Exercises

1. Suppose the transmission intensity that infective A exerts on susceptible B is described by the function

$$\psi(u) = \begin{cases} 0, & \text{for } 0 \le u < 1, \\ u - 1, & \text{for } 1 \le u < 2, \\ 2 - \frac{1}{2}u, & \text{for } 2 \le u < 4, \\ 0, & \text{for } u \ge 4, \end{cases} \tag{5.7}$$

where u is the time, in days, since A was infected.

(a) Sketch the graph of the transmission intensity function $\psi(u)$.

(b) What is the probability that A infects B within one day of being infected?

(c) Compute the probability that A infects B within two days of being infected.

(d) Compute the probability that B avoids infection by A.

(e) Find an expression for the probability that B is not infected by A within x days of the time of A's infection, where $1 < x < 2$.

(f) How soon after his infection must A be isolated so that the probability of B avoiding infection by A is at least 0.9?

2. Suppose A is the primary infective of a certain infectious disease. The transmission intensity A exerts on susceptible household partner B is described by the function $\psi(u)$ specified by (5.7). Independently, A exerts on susceptible neighbor C a transmission intensity described by $\frac{1}{4}\psi(u)$.

(a) Find the probability of event "*B and C avoid infection by A.*"

(b) Find the probability of event "*C is infected by A, but B is not.*"

3. Consider a community of uniformly mixing susceptibles. One of the susceptibles is infected by a contact with an outsider. Let u denote the time, in days, since the infection of this primary infective. Suppose the aggregated transmission intensity the primary infective exerts on the remaining susceptible community members is described by the function

$$\psi_{\Sigma}(u) = \begin{cases} 0, & \text{if } 0 \leq u < 1.5, \\ u - 1.5, & \text{if } 1.5 \leq u < 2.5, \\ 1, & \text{if } 2.5 \leq u < 4, \\ 3 - \frac{1}{2}u, & \text{if } 4 \leq u < 6, \\ 0, & \text{if } u \geq 6. \end{cases}$$

(a) Sketch the graph of the aggregated transmission intensity $\psi_{\Sigma}(u)$.

(b) Give the duration of the latent period.

(c) Give the duration of the infectious period.

(d) Find the initial reproduction number.

(e) Add the graph of the infectivity profile to your graph of part (a).

(f) Compute the initial reproduction number if *every* infected person is isolated exactly four days after being infected.

(g) Sketch the graph of the primary infective's infectivity profile if he is completely isolated exactly four days after being infected.

(h) How soon after their infection must infectives be isolated to ensure that an outbreak will be minor?

4. Consider a large community in which every household has two susceptibles. The community is free from a certain infectious disease when the infection is introduced by a community member who became infected by contacting an external infective.

Suppose the infectivity profile of the infection is given by

$$\omega(u) = \begin{cases} c, & \text{if } 1 \le u \le 5, \\ 0, & \text{otherwise,} \end{cases}$$

where c is a constant.
The within-household transmission intensity exerted by a primary household infective on his susceptible partner is described by the function $\omega(u)$. The aggregated transmission intensity an infective exerts, collectively, on individuals outside his household is described by the function $2\,\omega(u)$.

(a) Find the value of the constant c.

(b) Compute the probability that a primary household infective infects his susceptible household partner.

(c) Compute the initial household reproduction number R_{H}.

(d) Consider a public health intervention that isolates every infective u^* time units after his infection.

Compute the value u^*, such that this public health intervention achieves a post-intervention household reproduction number of $R^*_{\text{H}} = 1$.

5. Explain why the moving average of estimates given by Equation (5.2) produces a smoother estimated transmission intensity function.

6. Of a large uniformly mixing community of $n+1$ susceptible individuals, 80% are adults and 20% are children. Adult infectives have an infectivity profile

$$\omega_{\text{A}}(u) = \begin{cases} 0.5, & \text{if } 2 \le u \le 4, \\ 0, & \text{otherwise,} \end{cases}$$

and for children it is

$$\omega_{\text{C}}(u) = \begin{cases} 0.25, & \text{if } 1 \le u \le 5, \\ 0, & \text{otherwise.} \end{cases}$$

The transmission intensity between specific infective-susceptible pairs is summarized by the functions in the following table:

	Type of Susceptible	
	Adult	Child
Adult infective	$\frac{1}{n}\,\omega_{\text{A}}(u)$	$\frac{1.5}{n}\,\omega_{\text{A}}(u)$
Child infective	$\frac{2}{n}\,\omega_{\text{C}}(u)$	$\frac{3}{n}\,\omega_{\text{C}}(u)$

(a) Deduce the initial mean matrix for the number of offspring an infective generates during the initial stage of the outbreak.

(b) Find the initial reproduction number.

(c) Give circumstances under which isolating infected children at onset of symptoms ensures an outbreak is minor.

(d) Is it possible to ensure an outbreak is minor by early isolation of infected adults?

7. Consider a community of uniformly mixing susceptibles. Suppose the function given by

$$\psi_\Sigma(u) = \begin{cases} 0, & \text{if } 0 \le u < 1, \\ u-1, & \text{if } 1 \le u < 2, \\ 1, & \text{if } 2 \le u < 4, \\ 5-u, & \text{if } 4 \le u < 5, \\ 0, & \text{if } u \ge 6, \end{cases}$$

describes the aggregated transmission intensity exerted by the primary infective.

(a) Sketch the graph of the transmission intensity $\psi_\Sigma(u)$, $u \ge 0$.

(b) What is the mean number of individuals infected by the primary infective?

(c) What is the probability that the primary infective infects no one?

(d) Suppose a dose of antiviral drug is available that reduces an infective's infectivity by 50% for three days from the time it is taken.

(i) Determine when, ideally, the primary infective should commence taking the antiviral drug if the aim is to minimize the mean number of individuals he infects.

(ii) Is it certain that the outbreak will be minor if every infective takes a dose of the antiviral drug at the optimal time?

8. *A biology-based model for the infectivity profile*
Suppose a person is infected by ingesting a dose of pathogen during a contact with an infectious individual. Take the time of the infectious contact as $u = 0$ and measure time in days. Let $x(u)$ denote the size of the pathogen population within the host u days after the infectious contact. Denote the inherent growth rate of the pathogen population by λ = (birth rate) – (death rate), assumed to be constant. The response of the host's immune system is to decrease the growth rate by $\varphi(u)$, so that the size of the pathogen population within the host has a rate of increase given by

$$\frac{dx(u)}{du} = [\lambda - \varphi(u)]x(u)\,. \tag{5.8}$$

Note that λ is positive, while $\varphi(u)$ is initially zero and begins to increase when the immune system has detected the pathogen.

(a) Solve Equation (5.8) for $x(u)$ when

$$\varphi(u) = \begin{cases} 0, & \text{for } 0 \leq u \leq \tau, \\ \alpha(u-\tau)^{\gamma}, & \text{for } u > \tau. \end{cases}$$

(b) Suppose the infectivity profile of this infectious disease is given by $\omega(u) = c\,x(u)$, $u \geq 0$, where the constant c is such that the area under the graph of $\omega(u)$ is 1.

On the same graph, sketch the curves of the infectivity profiles given by $\omega(u)$ when

(i) $\tau = 2$, $\lambda = 2$, $\alpha = 2$ and $\gamma = 0.3$;

(ii) $\tau = 2$, $\lambda = 2$, $\alpha = 0.2$ and $\gamma = 2$.

9. *Progress of a household outbreak over time*

Consider a small household consisting of k homogeneous individuals who are susceptible to a certain infectious disease. Suppose one of them is infected by an external infectious contact. During the course of this household outbreak, the chance of infection from outside the household is assumed negligible compared to the chance of infection from within the household. Let the transmission intensity between an infective and a specific susceptible household partner be described by $\psi(u)$.

(a) With $k = 2$, let $N_2(t)$ denote the number infected within t days of the introduction of the infection into the household.

(i) Find expressions for probabilities $\Pr[N_2(t) = 1]$ and $\Pr[N_2(t) = 2]$ in terms of

$$\Psi(t) = \text{area under the graph of } \psi(u) \text{ between } u = 0 \text{ and } u = t.$$

(ii) Given that

$$\psi(u) = \begin{cases} 2, & \text{if } 1.5 \leq u \leq 4, \\ 0, & \text{otherwise}, \end{cases} \tag{5.9}$$

find $\nu_2(t) = \mathrm{E}[N_2(t)]$, the mean number infected in the household by time t, and sketch its graph.

(b) With $k = 3$, let $N_3(t)$ denote the number infected by time t. Assume that individuals avoid infection independently of each other.

(i) Find expressions for probabilities $\Pr[N_3(t) = 1]$, $\Pr[N_3(t) = 2]$ and $\Pr[N_3(t) = 3]$.

(ii) Given the transmission intensity described by the function (5.9) find $\nu_3(t) = \mathrm{E}[N_3(t)]$, the mean number infected by time t, and sketch its graph.

5.6 Supplementary material

5.6.1 Estimating the transmission intensity function

Consider the data on measles outbreaks in 232 households of size two described in Section 5.2. There are 45 households with only one case. For 187 households with two cases Figure 5.2 displays observations on n_6, n_7, $n_8, \ldots$, where n_j is taken to be the number of outbreaks in which a delay of j days is observed between the infection of the primary case and the infection of the secondary case. On the basis of these data we wish to estimate ψ_6, ψ_7, ψ_8, ... , where ψ_j denotes the value of the transmission intensity function on day j following the infection of the primary household case.

Using the probability (5.3) we derive the likelihood function of ψ_6, ψ_7, ψ_8, ... to be

$$\ell(\psi_6, \psi_7, \ldots) = \prod_{j=6} [\theta_j(1-\varepsilon_j)]^{n_j},$$

where $\varepsilon_j = \exp(-\psi_j)$ and

$$\theta_j = \begin{cases} 1 & \text{for } j = 6, \\ \prod_{i=6}^{j-1} \varepsilon_i & \text{for } j > 6. \end{cases}$$

We deduce that this likelihood function depends on ε_j only through

$$\varepsilon_j^{232-\sum_{i=6}^{j} n_i}(1-\varepsilon_j)^{n_j}.$$

As this has the same form as a likelihood function for Binomial data, we deduce that the maximum likelihood estimate of ε_j is

$$\hat{\varepsilon}_j = \frac{232 - \sum_{i=6}^{j} n_i}{232 - \sum_{i=6}^{j-1} n_i}.$$

The maximum likelihood estimate of ψ_j is therefore $\widehat{\psi}_j = -\ln(\hat{\varepsilon}_j)$.

Table 5.1: *Observed and fitted frequencies for time intervals between the detection of measles cases in households of size two*

Time interval	Observed frequency	Fitted frequency	Time interval	Observed frequency	Fitted frequency
6	4	4.8	14	15	11.9
7	11	7.8	15	6	7.2
8	5	11.8	16	3	3.2
9	25	24.1	17	1	2.0
10	37	35.4	18	3	1.8
11	38	34.7	19	0	0.7
12	26	24.4	20	0	0.3
13	12	15.9	21	1	0.5

Substituting the numerical values for the frequencies shown in Figure 5.2, which are given in Table 5.1, gives the maximum likelihood estimates of ε_j and ψ_j for $j = 6, 7, 8, \ldots$. The numerical values of these estimates are given in Table 5.2 and together they provide the estimated piecewise-constant transmission intensity function displayed in Figure 5.3.

Table 5.2: *Infectiousness function estimated from the times between measles cases in households of size two*

Interval	Estimates			Interval	Estimates		
j	$\hat{\varepsilon}_j$	$\widehat{\psi_j}$	$\overline{\psi}_j$	j	$\hat{\varepsilon}_j$	$\widehat{\psi_j}$	$\overline{\psi}_j$
6	.983	.017	.021	14	.797	.227	.178
7	.952	.049	.035	15	.898	.107	.125
8	.977	.023	.055	16	.943	.058	.061
9	.882	.125	.124	17	.980	.020	.040
10	.802	.220	.215	18	.939	.063	.037
11	.747	.292	.267	19	1.000	.000	.016
12	.768	.264	.243	20	1.000	.000	.006
13	.860	.150	.198	21	.978	.022	.011

5.6.2 Probability that a susceptible avoids infection

Consider a given pair of individuals, infective A and susceptible B. The function $\psi(u)$, $u \geq 0$, describes the transmission intensity that A exerts on B, in the period following the infection of A. Our aim is to find an expression for the probability that B avoids being infected by A over the time interval $0 \leq u \leq t$.

Construct a partition of the time interval $(0, t)$ by the k increments between time points $u_0, u_1, u_2, \ldots, u_k$, where $0 = u_0 < u_1 < u_2 < \cdots < u_k = t$. Let $\delta_j = u_j - u_{j-1}$, for $j = 1, 2, \ldots, k$. Suppose k is large and each δ_j is small. The conditional probability that B avoids infection in the time increment (u_{j-1}, u_j), given that B was not infected by A prior to time u_{j-1}, is approximately

$$1 - \psi(u_{j-1})\,\delta_j \;\approx\; \exp\left[-\psi(u_{j-1})\,\delta_j\right].$$

For B to avoid infection by A in the time interval $(0, t)$ he must avoid infection in every one of the above k time increments. Therefore the probability that B avoids infection by A over the time interval $0 \leq u \leq t$ is approximated by

$$\prod_{j=1}^{k} \exp\left[-\psi(u_{j-1})\,\delta_j\right] = \exp\left[-\sum_{j=1}^{k} \psi(u_{j-1})\,\delta_j\right].$$

As we let $k \to \infty$, in a way so that every $\delta_j \to 0$, this gives

$$\Pr(\text{B is not infected by A by time } t) = \exp\left[-\Psi(t)\right],$$

where

$$\begin{aligned}\Psi(t) &= \text{area under the curve } \psi(u) \text{ between } u = 0 \text{ and } u = t,\\ &= \int_0^t \psi(u)\, du.\end{aligned}$$

5.6.3 Transmission in a uniformly mixing community

Mean number of offspring

Consider a primary infective who exerts a small transmission intensity on each community susceptible. Let $\psi_\Sigma(u)$ be the sum of these intensities at time u after the infection of the primary infective. As in Section 5.6.2, construct a partition $0 = u_0, u_1, u_2, \ldots, u_k = t$ of the time interval $(0, t)$, where k is large and each $\delta_j = u_j - u_{j-1}$ is small. The probability that this primary infective makes an infectious contact in the short time increment (u_{j-1}, u_j) is approximately given by

$$\Pr(\text{he infects 1 person}) = \psi_\Sigma(u_{j-1})\,\delta_j = 1 - \Pr(\text{he infects no one}), \quad (5.10)$$

with the approximation improving as δ_j becomes small.

The mean number of individuals infected by the primary infective in the time increment (u_{j-1}, u_j) is therefore approximately

$$0 \times [1 - \psi_\Sigma(u_{j-1})\,\delta_j] \; + \; 1 \times \psi_\Sigma(u_{j-1})\,\delta_j \; = \; \psi_\Sigma(u_{j-1})\,\delta_j.$$

The number of individuals infected by the primary infective over the time interval from $u = 0$ to $u = t$ is obtained by summing the mean number infected in each of the time increments of the partition. It follows that the mean number of offspring the primary infective produces in the time interval $(0, t)$ is given by

$$\sum_{j=1}^{k} \psi_\Sigma(u_{j-1})\,\delta_j \; = \; \int_0^t \psi_\Sigma(u)\, du \; = \; \Psi_\Sigma(t).$$

The mean number of offspring the primary infective has over his entire infectious period is the initial reproduction number given by

$$R \; = \; \int_{u_{\mathrm{L}}}^{u_{\mathrm{L}} + u_{\mathrm{I}}} \psi_\Sigma(u)\, du \; = \; \Psi_\Sigma(u_{\mathrm{L}} + u_{\mathrm{I}}),$$

where u_{L} is the duration of the latent period and u_{I} is the duration of the infectious period.

This shows that, in this setting, the initial reproduction number is given by the total area under the graph of the aggregated transmission intensity function.

The Poisson distribution is a natural baseline offspring distribution

We now find the distribution of the number of individuals primary infective A infects, assuming that the following is true:

(i) the community has a large number of susceptibles,

(ii) infective A mixes uniformly with all susceptibles,

(iii) the transmission intensity exerted by A, collectively on all susceptibles, is described by aggregated transmission intensity function $\psi_{\Sigma}(u)$, where u is the time since the infection of A.

Our approach is to find the probability generating function and then recognize the corresponding probability distribution.

Again we use the partition $0 = u_0, u_1, u_2, \ldots, u_k = t$ of the time interval $(0, t)$, where k is large and each $\delta_j = u_j - u_{j-1}$ is small. Using Equation (5.10) we find the probability generation function for X_j, the number of infections generated by infective A in the time increment (u_{j-1}, u_j), to be approximately

$$\mathrm{E}\left(z^{X_j}\right) = [1 - \psi_{\Sigma}(u_{j-1})\delta_j] + \psi_{\Sigma}(u_{j-1})\delta_j z \approx \exp\left[(z-1)\psi_{\Sigma}(u_{j-1})\,\delta_j\right],$$

with the approximation improving as the δ_j become smaller. We deduce that the probability generating function of the number of individuals primary infective A infects in the time interval $(0, t)$ is given by

$$\begin{aligned} \mathrm{E}\left(z^{\sum_{j=1}^{k} X_j}\right) &\approx \exp\left[(z-1)\sum_{j=1}^{k}\psi_{\Sigma}(u_{j-1})\,\delta_j\right], \\ &\approx \exp\left[(z-1)\Psi_{\Sigma}(t)\right], \end{aligned} \qquad (5.11)$$

where

$$\Psi_{\Sigma}(t) = \text{area under the curve } \psi_{\Sigma}(u) \text{ between } u = 0 \text{ and } u = t.$$

The expression on the right-hand side of (5.11) is recognized as the probability generating function of the Poisson distribution with mean $\Psi_{\Sigma}(t)$. We conclude that, under the stated assumptions, the number of community members infected by the primary infective A over the time interval from his infection (at time $u = 0$) until t time units later has a Poisson distribution with mean $\Psi_{\Sigma}(t) = \int_0^t \psi_{\Sigma}(u)\,du$.

By substituting the particular time $t = u_{\mathrm{L}} + u_{\mathrm{I}}$, where u_{L} is the duration of the latent period and u_{I} is the duration of the infectious period, we conclude that the offspring distribution of the primary infective is Poisson with mean $\mu = \int_{u_{\mathrm{L}}}^{u_{\mathrm{L}}+u_{\mathrm{I}}} \psi_{\Sigma}(u)\,du$.

This demonstrates that the Poisson offspring distribution applies in a situation where each infective, during the early stages of an outbreak, has exactly the same aggregated transmission intensity function. We can therefore view the Poisson offspring distribution as a benchmark offspring distribution.

Other offspring distributions arise when we allow for unpredictable, i.e., random, differences in the transmission intensity function of infectives. For example, there can be random differences in the rate at which hosts shed pathogen, the duration for which they shed pathogen or the mixing rates of individuals.

5.7 Bibliographic notes

Although fundamental, the notion of a transmission intensity function has received limited attention in the literature. Becker (1989, Chapter 3) introduced it under the name of *infectiousness function*, while Jewell and Shiboski (1990) use the term *infectivity function* in their work on estimating the function from data on the transmission of HIV between partners.

CHAPTER 6

Partially effective vaccines

The preferred method for controlling an infectious disease is to vaccinate as many individuals as possible with a vaccine that is safe, fully protective and provides immunity that does not wane. While some vaccines, such as the measles vaccine, come close to this ideal, most are less effective. Modeling needs to allow for vaccines that are not fully protective.

To have a chance of being adopted a candidate vaccine must be safe and able to reduce one or more of the following:

a. an individual's chance of being infected,
b. severity of illness in a vaccinee who acquires a breakthrough infection,
c. infectivity of a vaccinee who acquires a breakthrough infection.

We focus our discussion on the ability of the vaccine to reduce transmission of the infectious disease. That is, our emphasis is on the extent to which a vaccine reduces susceptibility and infectivity in vaccinees. These reductions are reflected in a model by introducing a corresponding reduction in the transmission intensity between individuals.

In this chapter we determine conditions under which a mass immunization campaign prevents epidemics when the vaccine is partially effective. Unless stated otherwise, we assume that an individual's mixing rate is unaltered by vaccination.

6.1 Vaccine effect on transmission between individuals

To describe how a partially effective vaccine might change the transmission intensity between a pair of individuals, consider infective A and susceptible B. Let $\psi(u)$ be the function describing the transmission intensity between A and B when neither of them is vaccinated, nor has acquired immunity from a previous infection. Recall, from Equation (5.4), that

$$\Pr(B \text{ avoids infection by } A) \;=\; \exp(-\Psi) \;=\; q, \text{ say}, \qquad (6.1)$$

where Ψ is the total area under the graph of transmission intensity function $\psi(u)$.

6.1.1 The susceptible is a vaccinee

Consider first how the transmission intensity differs from $\psi(u)$ when susceptible B is a vaccinee, but infective A is not.

We model the effect of the vaccine on susceptibility by changing the probability of the infection being transmitted during a small time increment $(u, u + \delta)$ by a factor a when the contacted susceptible is a vaccinee. That is, the probability $\psi(u)\,\delta$ in Equation (5.1) becomes $a\psi(u)\,\delta$. The vaccine provides full protection against infection when $a = 0$ and offers no protection when $a = 1$. In practice, a is likely to have a value between 0 and 1.

This change in the chance of transmission applies independently to every small time increment. As a consequence, the transmission intensity between A and B changes from $\psi(u)$ to $a\psi(u)$ for all $u \geq 0$ when the vaccination status of B changes from unvaccinated to vaccinated.

Graphs (a) and (b) of Figure 6.1 illustrate this form of change to the transmission intensity, where (a) is the graph of $\psi(u)$ and (b) is the graph of $a\psi(u)$ with $a = 0.2$.

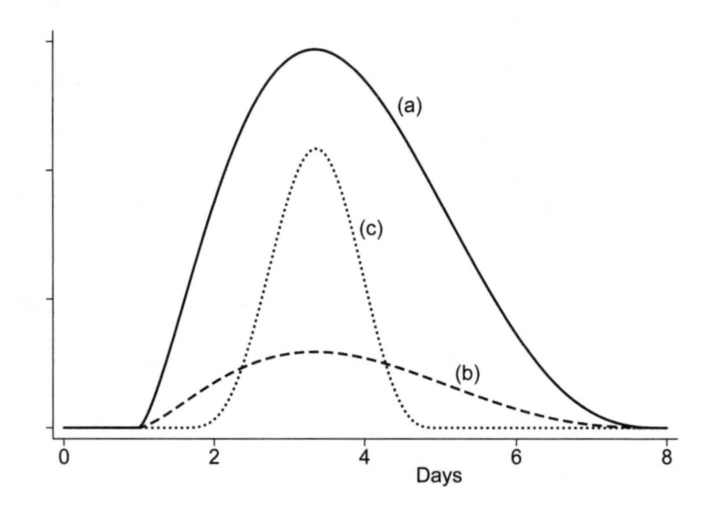

Figure 6.1 *Illustrative graphs of the transmission intensity between an infective A and a susceptible B. Graph (a) shows the transmission intensity when both individuals are unvaccinated and graphs (b) and (c) illustrate possible vaccine effects on this transmission intensity. Vaccine effect (b) is a proportionate reduction in the transmission intensity at every time point. Vaccine effect (c) illustrates a reduction that includes a longer latent period and a shorter infectious period.*

By changing the transmission intensity function from $\psi(u)$ to $a\psi(u)$ we find, from Equation (6.1), that

$$\Pr(B \text{ avoids infection by } A) \;=\; \exp(-a\Psi) \;=\; q^a$$

when susceptible B is a vaccinee, but infective A is not. A comparison with (6.1) shows how this probability is changed by changing the vaccination status of B.

6.1.2 *The infective is a vaccinee*

Different vaccines affect the infectivity of a vaccinee with a breakthrough infection in different ways. To quantify this vaccine effect it helps to think of the transmission intensity between an unvaccinated infective-susceptible pair in the form $\psi(u) = \beta\omega(u)$. Here $\omega(u)$ is the infectivity profile, which reflects the *pattern* of the amount of pathogen shed by the infective over time. The constant β is determined by the overall amount of pathogen shed by the infective, the ease with which the susceptible ingests the pathogen and the social contact rate between them.

Suppose now that A is a vaccinee who acquires a breakthrough infection and susceptible B is unvaccinated. The transmission intensity between such a pair can differ from $\psi(u) = \beta\omega(u)$ in many different ways, depending on the nature of the immune response induced by the vaccine. To illustrate plausible changes it is useful to write the changed transmission intensity between such a pair of individuals as $\psi^*(u) = b\beta\omega^*(u)$, where $\omega^*(u)$ reflects any change in the infectivity profile of A as a result of being vaccinated and the constant b reflects the overall change in infectivity.

The graphs in Figure 6.1 illustrate two possible forms for the way vaccination of A might alter the transmission intensity. Let Curve (a) in Figure 6.1 be the graph of $\psi(u) = \beta\omega(u)$, the intensity when neither A nor B is vaccinated. Curves (b) and (c) illustrate two possible vaccine effects on infectivity.

In Curve (b) the altered transmission intensity has the form $\psi^*(u) = 0.2\psi(u) = 0.2\beta\omega(u)$. In words, vaccinating A induced the same proportionate reduction in his infectivity at every time point following the infection of A. This vaccine response does not change the infectivity profile of A, but it does reduce the overall infectivity substantially.

Curve (c) illustrates a situation where vaccination changes the transmission intensity exerted by individual A in a way that includes an increase in the duration of the latent period and a decrease in the duration of the infectious period. The infectivity profile is changed by this vaccine response.

Earlier we used Curve (b) of Figure 6.1 to illustrate a possible effect of vaccination on susceptibility and now, separately, we have used it to illustrate a proportionate reduction in infectivity. Either effect, or a combination of two such effects, can lead to transmission intensity (b).

By changing the transmission intensity function from $\psi(u) = \beta\omega(u)$ to $\psi^*(u) = b\beta\omega^*(u)$ we find, from Equation (6.1), that

$$\Pr(B \text{ avoids infection by } A) \;=\; \exp\left(-b\Psi\right) \;=\; q^b$$

when infective A is a vaccinee, but susceptible B is not. A comparison with (6.1) shows how this probability is changed by changing the vaccination status of A.

6.1.3 Both individuals are vaccinees

Suppose now that susceptibles A and B are vaccinees, and A acquires a breakthrough infection. The expression for the transmission intensity between them must then include the effect of the vaccine on the infectivity of A *and* its effect on the susceptibility of B. The resulting transmission intensity might then be expressed by $ab\beta\omega^*(u)$, which assumes that the susceptibility effect of the vaccine does not depend on the vaccination status of the infective.

By changing the transmission intensity function from $\psi(u) = \beta\omega(u)$ to $\psi^*(u) = ab\beta\omega^*(u)$ we find, from Equation (6.1), that

$$\Pr(B \text{ avoids infection by } A) \;=\; \exp(-ab\Psi) \;=\; q^{ab}$$

when A and B are vaccinees. A comparison with (6.1) reveals how this probability is changed by vaccinating both A and B.

Table 6.1 summarizes the effect of vaccination on the transmission intensity for the four possible vaccination status combinations.

Table 6.1: *Transmission intensity u days after A is infected*

		Susceptible B	
		unvaccinated	vaccinated
Infective A	unvaccinated	$\beta\omega(u)$	$a\beta\omega(u)$
Infective A	vaccinated	$b\beta\omega^*(u)$	$ab\beta\omega^*(u)$

6.2 Impact of mass immunization on the reproduction number

We illustrate how these vaccine effects impact on the reproduction number in two community settings.

6.2.1 A community of homogeneous individuals who mix uniformly

Consider a large community consisting of $n+1$ homogeneous susceptibles who mix uniformly. Suppose the basic reproduction number for a certain infectious disease in this community is R_0.

When a fraction v of community members is vaccinated with a partially effective vaccine we have two types of individual. Unvaccinated individuals are Type 1 and vaccinated individuals are Type 2. The post-campaign reproduction number is determined by the type-specific mean number of offspring.

In this setting the transmission intensity between any given infective-susceptiple pair depends on their types. Using vaccine effects of the form shown in Table 6.1, with $\beta\omega(u) = \frac{1}{n}R_0\omega(u)$, the matrix of type-specific means number of offspring is given by

$$\begin{pmatrix} \mu_{11}^* & \mu_{12}^* \\ \mu_{21}^* & \mu_{22}^* \end{pmatrix} = \begin{pmatrix} \tilde{v}R_0 & avR_0 \\ b\tilde{v}R_0 & abvR_0 \end{pmatrix}, \tag{6.2}$$

where R_0 is the basic reproduction number and $\tilde{v} = 1 - v$. The asterisks on the left-hand side of Equation (6.2) are there to remind us that these are the values of the type-specific means *after* the immunization campaign. By substituting the elements of this mean matrix into Equation (4.2) we obtain the post-campaign reproduction number

$$R_v^* = \tilde{v}R_0 + vR_1 = [1 - (1 - ab)v]R_0,$$

where $R_1 = abR_0$ is the reproduction number when all individuals are vaccinated.

Note that a is the factor by which the vaccine lowers the probability of infection during every contact a vaccinated susceptible has with an infective, while b is the factor by which vaccination reduces the total area under the function describing the transmission intensity exerted by a vaccinee with a breakthrough infection compared to the corresponding area for an unvaccinated infective. More intuitively, b is the factor by which the total infectivity of an individual is reduced by being vaccinated, in the event that he becomes infected.

The term $(1 - ab)v$, in the expression for R_v^*, is the immunity coverage when either the vaccine is fully protective ($a = 0$) or the vaccine fully prevents infectivity in the vaccinee ($b = 0$). More generally, we can view $(1-ab)v$ as the fraction of *community immunity* achieved. The factor $1 - ab$ can be viewed as a measure of the *vaccine efficacy for reducing transmission.* It is interesting to observe that the susceptibility effect a and the infectivity effect b are interchangeable, as far as vaccine effect on the reproduction number is concerned.

The reproduction number is $R_1 = abR_0$ when everyone is vaccinated. We deduce that $R_1 < 1$ only if $ab < 1/R_0$. That is, the vaccine can only prevent epidemics when $ab < 1/R_0$. When this inequality holds, the critical vaccination coverage is

$$v^\dagger = \frac{R_0 - 1}{R_0 - R_1} = \frac{1 - 1/R_0}{1 - ab}.$$

6.2.2 *A community of households*

To illustrate how immunization with a partially effective vaccine changes the household reproduction number we consider a community consisting of a large number of households of size 2 with all members susceptible. For this setting the basic household reproduction number is

$$R_{\text{H0}} = \mu\nu_2,$$

where μ is the mean number of individuals a primary infective infects outside his household and $\nu_2 = 1 + \tilde{q}$ is the mean size of an outbreak that evolves independently in a household with one primary infective who has exactly one susceptible household partner. Here $\tilde{q}$ is the probability that the primary household infective infects his household partner.

Suppose a mass immunization campaign vaccinates both members in a fraction v of the households with a partially effective vaccine. We again need to allow for two types of individual, namely unvaccinated (Type 1) and vaccinated (Type 2) individuals. As we have a community with a household setting we need to consider the effect of the immunization campaign on between-household transmission and on within-household transmission.

In Section 6.6, by considering how the immunization campaign changes the values of μ and ν_2, we find what the elements of the type-specific mean matrix (4.4) are after the immunization campaign. Substituting these into Equation (4.5) gives the post-campaign reproduction number

$$R_{\mathrm{H}}^* = \tilde{v}R_{\mathrm{H0}} - vR_{\mathrm{H1}},$$

where $\tilde{v} = 1 - v$ and $R_{\mathrm{H1}} = ab\mu(2 - q^{ab})$ is the reproduction number when the vaccination coverage is 100%.

Epidemics are prevented when $R_{\mathrm{H1}} < 1$ and so the vaccine can prevent epidemics only when the product ab is small enough to make $ab\mu(2-q^{ab}) < 1$. When this is so, the critical vaccination coverage is given by

$$v^{\dagger} = \frac{R_{\mathrm{H0}} - 1}{R_{\mathrm{H0}} - R_{\mathrm{H1}}}.$$

Note that again the susceptibility effect a and the infectivity effect b are interchangeable in this expression.

6.3 Estimating vaccine effects

To estimate a, the vaccine effect on susceptibility, and b, the vaccine effect on infectivity, one should ideally observe, for each infection, the vaccination status of both the infector and the individual infected. In practice the source of an infection is often not observed. Fortunately, data on outbreaks in households contain at least implicit information about the source of an infection.

To illustrate how data on the size of household outbreaks can be used to estimate a and b we consider frequency data for outbreaks in households that include two susceptibles. It is assumed that the vaccination status of household members is also observed. This method of estimation is readily extended to outbreak data on households with more susceptibles.

The probability for each possible type of household outbreak is given in Table 6.2, where $q = \exp(-\beta_{\mathrm{H}})$. Suppose we have observed each of the

Table 6.2: *Probability for each possible household outbreak*

Vaccination status		Outbreak size	
Primary infective	Household partner	1	2
unvaccinated	unvaccinated	q	$1-q$
unvaccinated	vaccinated	q^a	$1-q^a$
vaccinated	unvaccinated	q^b	$1-q^b$
vaccinated	vaccinated	q^{ab}	$1-q^{ab}$

possible outbreaks a number of times, with the frequencies shown in Table 6.3.

The likelihood function corresponding to such frequency data is given by

$$\ell(a, b, q) = q^{n_1}(1-q)^{n_2} q^{an_3}(1-q^a)^{n_4} q^{bn_5}(1-q^b)^{n_6} q^{abn_7}(1-q^{ab})^{n_8}.$$

Substituting the numerical frequencies into the likelihood function and finding the values of a, b and q at which this function assumes its maximum value gives the maximum likelihood estimates of a, b and q. In the maximization each of a, b and q is restricted to take a value between 0 and 1, assuming that the vaccine does not increase susceptibility, nor increase infectivity. Standard large sample likelihood methods provide standard errors for these estimates.

Table 6.3: *Frequency data for possible household outbreaks*

Vaccination status		Outbreak size	
Primary infective	Household partner	1	2
unvaccinated	unvaccinated	n_1	n_2
unvaccinated	vaccinated	n_3	n_4
vaccinated	unvaccinated	n_5	n_6
vaccinated	vaccinated	n_7	n_8

6.4 Discussion

The effects of a partially effective vaccine on susceptibility and infectivity have been modeled in terms of two constants, a and b. They represent the fraction by which susceptibility and infectivity are reduced, respectively, but with different interpretations. It is useful to explain why the form of the impact of these two vaccine effects on transmission is similar despite the difference in their interpretations.

Differences in interpretation: Susceptibility effect a is the factor by which the per-contact probability of transmission is changed when the vaccination status of the contacted individual is changed from unvaccinated to vaccinated. This change in vaccination status leaves the infectivity profile between the pair of individuals unchanged. Infectivity effect b is the factor by which the total potential to infect a given individual is changed by changing the vaccination status of the infective from unvaccinated to vaccinated, as measured by the *total* area under the graph of the transmission intensity between them. The change in vaccination status of the infective can change the infectivity profile between the pair of individuals substantially.

Similarity in impacts: Let q be the probability that a susceptible avoids being infected by a given infective over the infective's entire infectious period, when both are unvaccinated individuals. This probability changes to

$$\begin{cases} q^a & \text{when the susceptible's status is changed to vaccinated,} \\ q^b & \text{when the infective's status is changed to vaccinated.} \end{cases}$$

The similar form of the impact of the two different vaccine effects on the probability q is explained by the fact that the probability of avoiding infection is determined by the total area under the graph of the transmission intensity between the two individuals, as in Equation (6.1). The vaccine effect on infectivity, b, is defined explicitly in terms of the factor by which this area is changed by changing the vaccination status of the infective. The vaccine effect on susceptibility, a, is defined differently, but its definition can be used to show that a equals the factor by which the total area under the graph of the transmission intensity between the two individuals is changed by changing the vaccination status of the susceptible. This explains the similarity of the *form* of the vaccine effect. In practice the values of a and b can be quite different.

The description of vaccine effects on susceptibility and infectivity given in this chapter assumes that every vaccinee has the same vaccine response. This assumption can be relaxed to allow a random vaccine response to be allocated to each vaccinee. Exercise 4 in Section 6.5 gives a simple illustration of this.

The underlying assumption that individuals do not change their mixing behavior when they are vaccinated is something we need to be aware of. For example, suppose an individual is vaccinated with a vaccine that reduces the per-contact risk of acquiring a sexually transmissible disease, but is not fully protective. The susceptibility of a vaccinee might actually increase if, assuming he is protected, he becomes less discriminatory in his choice of sexual partners, engages in unsafe sex practices and has casual sex more frequently.

As we have modeled it, the effect of a vaccine is to reduce susceptibility and infectivity in the vaccinee by constant amounts a and b, respectively. Other vaccine effects are possible. For example, a and b might vary among vaccinees. An extreme case of this is when vaccinations occasionally fail to provide any protection to the vaccinee. Exercise 4, below, illustrates how such a vaccine effect can be accommodated.

6.5 Exercises

1. The transmission intensity that an unvaccinated infective A exerts on a certain unvaccinated susceptible B is described by the function

$$\psi(u) = \begin{cases} 0, & \text{for } 0 \leq u < 1, \\ u - 1, & \text{for } 1 \leq u < 2, \\ 2 - \frac{1}{2}u, & \text{for } 2 \leq u < 4, \\ 0, & \text{for } u \geq 4, \end{cases}$$

   where u is the time, in days, since A was infected.

   Consider now, separately, a change in the vaccination status of individuals A and B, with a newly developed vaccine.

   The vaccine's effect on susceptibility is to halve the per-contact probability that the infection is transmitted to B when the vaccination status of B is changed to "vaccinated."

   The effect of this vaccine on infectivity is described by $\psi(u)$, the transmission intensity between A and B, changing to

$$\psi^*(u) = \begin{cases} 0, & \text{for } 0 \leq u < 1, \\ \frac{1}{2}(u - 1), & \text{for } 1 \leq u < 2, \\ \frac{1}{2}(3 - u), & \text{for } 2 \leq u < 3, \\ 0, & \text{for } u \geq 3, \end{cases}$$

   when the vaccination status of A is changed to "vaccinated," while the vaccination status of susceptible B remains "unvaccinated."

   (a) Using the notation of Table 6.1, determine the values of a and b, and the forms of the profiles $\omega(u)$ and $\omega^*(u)$.

   (b) Specify the effect of the vaccine on the duration of

      (i) the latent period, and

      (ii) the infectious period.

   (c) Determine how the probability of event "A infects B" changes as their vaccination status changes from "both unvaccinated" to

      (i) A unvaccinated, B vaccinated,

      (ii) A vaccinated, B unvaccinated,

      (iii) both vaccinated.

2. An immunization campaign is to be conducted against a certain infectious disease in a community consisting of homogeneous individuals who are susceptible and mix uniformly. The basic reproduction number for

the infectious disease in this community is 2.0. Three candidate vaccines are available, with the following vaccine effects:

	Susceptibility effect, a	Infectivity effect, b
Vaccine 1	0.5	0.5
Vaccine 2	0.7	0.3
Vaccine 3	0.9	0.1

(a) Which vaccine achieves the lowest post-campaign effective reproduction number when everyone is vaccinated?

(b) In practice, uptake of a vaccine depends on the level of protection it offers the vaccinee against infection. It is estimated that the achievable coverage is 70%, 50% and 30% for Vaccine 1, 2 and 3, respectively.

Taking achievable coverages into account, which vaccine should be adopted for the proposed immunization campaign?

3. Consider a community in which all households consist of two individuals who are susceptible to a certain infectious disease. The household reproduction number for this infectious disease is

$$R_{\text{H0}} = \mu\,[1 + \tilde{q}],$$

where μ is the mean number of individuals a primary infective infects outside his household and $\tilde{q}$ is the probability that a primary household infective infects his household partner. In order to reduce within-household transmission, in the event of an outbreak, a mass immunization campaign is conducted with a vaccine that is partially effective. Susceptibles are selected for vaccination sequentially, by selecting exactly one individual from a household that still has two unvaccinated household members. In this way, a fraction v of individuals is vaccinated, where $v \leq \frac{1}{2}$.

(a) Find an expression for the post-campaign household reproduction number.

(b) Specify circumstances under which this campaign is able to prevent epidemics.

(c) Given circumstances under which this campaign strategy is able to prevent epidemics, what is the critical vaccination coverage?

4. Consider a community consisting of homogeneous individuals who mix uniformly. All are susceptible to being infected with a certain infectious disease. Let R_0 be the basic reproduction number of the infectious disease in this community. An immunization campaign, selecting individuals randomly, achieves a community coverage of v. The vaccine used in this campaign fails, i.e., induces no effect on susceptibility and no effect on infectivity, in a fraction f of vaccinees. A successful vaccination induces a susceptibility effect a and an infectivity effect b.

Use a model with two types to find an expression for

(a) the post-campaign reproduction number R^*, and

(b) the critical vaccination coverage, if it exists.

5. Consider a household consisting of a newly infected individual A and his household partner B. Suppose the vaccine for this infection has susceptibility effect a and infectivity effect also equal to a.

   We deduce that the two vaccination status scenarios (A vaccinated, B unvaccinated) and (A unvaccinated, B vaccinated) give the same value for Pr(B avoids infection by A).

   Explain then why these two scenarios could give quite different values for Pr(B is not infected by A within 3 days of A's time of infection).

6.6 Supplementary material

Effect of mass vaccination on the household reproduction number

Consider the early stage of an outbreak of an infectious disease that has been introduced into a large community of households. Each household has two homogeneous susceptibles. An immunization campaign vaccinates both susceptible members in a fraction v of households with a partially effective vaccine. Post-campaign we have two types of individual, namely unvaccinated (Type 1) and vaccinated (Type 2) individuals.

To determine how the campaign impacts on the household reproduction number we look at the changes to between-household transmission and, separately, changes to within-household transmission.

(a) Vaccine effect on between-household transmission

In the notation of Section 4.3, we deduce that the type-specific mean number of community members an infective infects outside his household is

$$\begin{pmatrix} \mu_{11}^* & \mu_{12}^* \\ \mu_{21}^* & \mu_{22}^* \end{pmatrix} = \begin{pmatrix} \mu\tilde{v} & a\mu v \\ b\mu\tilde{v} & ab\mu v \end{pmatrix},$$

where the asterisks indicate that these are post-campaign means and $\tilde{v} = 1 - v$.

(b) Vaccine effect on within-household transmission

We can translate the vaccine effects as described by the elements of Table 6.1 to transmission within households by using Equation (5.4). For two household partners, infective A and susceptible B, the probability that B avoids infection by A depends on the vaccination status of both A and B. Let the transmission intensity between A and B be as in Table 6.1 with β_{H} in place of β, to remind us that we are considering a transmission intensity between two household partners. In this notation Table 6.4 gives the probability of B avoiding infection by his household partner, for the four possible vaccination status combinations of A and B. Note that the vaccine effects a and b enter the probability expressions in the exponent.

Table 6.4: *Probability of avoiding infection by a household partner*

		Susceptible household partner B	
		unvaccinated	vaccinated
Infective A	unvaccinated	$\exp(-\beta_{\text{H}}) = q$	$\exp(-a\beta_{\text{H}}) = q^a$
Infective A	vaccinated	$\exp(-b\beta_{\text{H}}) = q^b$	$\exp(-ab\beta_{\text{H}}) = q^{ab}$

With the assumed form of immunization both members of each household are of the same type. Therefore, the type-specific mean number infected in a household outbreak, following the immunization campaign, is

$$\begin{pmatrix} \nu_{11}^* & \nu_{12}^* \\ \nu_{21}^* & \nu_{22}^* \end{pmatrix} = \begin{pmatrix} 2-q & 0 \\ 0 & 2-q^{ab} \end{pmatrix}.$$

(c) Combining changes to between- and within-household transmission

Substituting these terms into the expressions for the four elements of the mean matrix (4.4) we find the mean matrix

$$\begin{pmatrix} m_{11}^* & m_{12}^* \\ m_{21}^* & m_{22}^* \end{pmatrix} = \begin{pmatrix} \mu\tilde{v}(2-q) & a\mu v(2-q^{ab}) \\ b\mu\tilde{v}(2-q) & ab\mu v(2-q^{ab}) \end{pmatrix}.$$

With these elements Equation (4.2) gives the post-campaign household reproduction number

$$R_{\text{H}}^* = \mu\tilde{v}(2-q) + ab\mu v(2-q^{ab}) = \tilde{v}R_{\text{H0}} + vR_{\text{H1}},$$

where $R_{\text{H0}} = \mu(2-q)$ is the reproduction number in the absence of vaccination and $R_{\text{H1}} = ab\mu(2-q^{ab})$ is the household reproduction number when the vaccination coverage is 100%.

6.7 Bibliographic notes

Our formulation of the effect of vaccination on susceptibility and infectivity is often referred to as a *leaky* response. Another type of response is the *all-or-nothing* response, which allows for vaccine failures as Exercise 4 of Section 6.5. Becker and Starczak (1998) allow the vaccine response to be random, which includes the leaky response and the all-or-nothing response as special cases.

The review by Halloran et al. (1997) and the book by Halloran et al. (2010) give a comprehensive discussion of a wide range of vaccine responses.

CHAPTER 7

Social distancing

For some infectious diseases, including newly emerged infections, no safe, effective vaccine exists. It is then necessary to respond to a new outbreak with temporary measures, such as promoting social distancing and administering antiviral drugs, if available. Much consideration is given to such measures when developing preparedness plans for pandemic influenza, for example. In this chapter we illustrate how to incorporate the effect of social distancing into models.

7.1 What is social distancing?

An outbreak of an infectious disease is progressed by close contacts between infectious and susceptible individuals. Reducing the frequency of such contacts is therefore a natural way to slow, and possibly limit, the progress of an outbreak. Social distancing measures are public health interventions that aim to reduce the frequency of close contacts between people. When possible, these measures focus on individuals who have been exposed to the infectious disease and individuals considered at highest risk of being exposed.

There is a vast range of social distancing measures. Some target all community members, some target specific types of individual and some target infectives and their households. Social distancing measures include:

(i) Encourage individuals to spend less time in public places such as shopping malls and movie theaters. This has the attraction of being an instantaneous response, although compliance is often an issue.

(ii) Isolate infectives at onset of symptoms. This inconveniences primarily individuals with a confirmed infection.

(iii) Quarantine infected households. This focuses on confirmed cases and individuals who are most exposed to them.

(iv) Close schools. An option often considered when children are the main transmitters of the infection. It presents difficulties for working parents.

(v) Ban mass gatherings such as sporting events and concerts. This can avoid multiple infections, but is often resisted on commercial grounds.

People are reluctant to accept changes to their lifestyle without compelling reasons to do so. It is therefore essential to have convincing arguments to support the introduction of social distancing measures. An assessment of the likely effectiveness and benefits of social distancing measures based on modeling can help to provide persuasive arguments for their introduction.

We now illustrate how the effect of some of these measures can be incorporated into infectious disease models.

7.2 Reduced mixing

Suppose a new infectious disease emerges in a uniformly mixing community consisting of $n+1$ susceptibles and the public health authority issues guidelines for social distancing. In response, a fraction f of individuals reduces its mixing with community members by a factor a. For example, they reduce the time they spend in public places, such as shopping malls, to a fraction a of their usual time. We then have two types of individual, namely non-responders (Type 1) and responders (Type 2). Table 7.1 gives the changes to the pairwise transmission intensities when the transmission intensity between two individuals who have not changed their mixing rate is given by $\frac{1}{n}\psi(u)$, $u \geq 0$.

Table 7.1: *Infection intensity between infective A and specific susceptible B, u days after the infection of A*

		Susceptible B	
		non-responder	responder
Infective A	non-responder	$\frac{1}{n}\psi(u)$	$\frac{a}{n}\psi(u)$
Infective A	responder	$\frac{a}{n}\psi(u)$	$\frac{a^2}{n}\psi(u)$

The form of the bottom right-hand element in this table, namely $\frac{a^2}{n}\psi(u)$, arises under the assumption that responders choose times to mix in public locations independently. The graphs in Figure 7.1 show a form for the three transmission intensities of Table 7.1 when a takes the value 0.5.

The associated mean matrix for the number of infections by these two types of infective, during the early stage of the outbreak, is

$$\begin{pmatrix} \mu_{11}^* & \mu_{12}^* \\ \mu_{21}^* & \mu_{22}^* \end{pmatrix} = \begin{pmatrix} \tilde{f}R_0 & afR_0 \\ a\tilde{f}R_0 & a^2fR_0 \end{pmatrix}, \tag{7.1}$$

where $\tilde{f} = 1 - f$ and R_0 = the area under the aggregated transmission intensity function $\psi(u)$, $u \geq 0$. Again, the asterisks are there to remind us that these type-specific means are the post-intervention means. Substituting the elements of mean matrix (7.1) into Equation (4.2) we find the post-intervention reproduction number for this community to be

$$R^* = [1 - (1 - a^2)f]R_0 = \tilde{f}R_0 + fR_1,$$

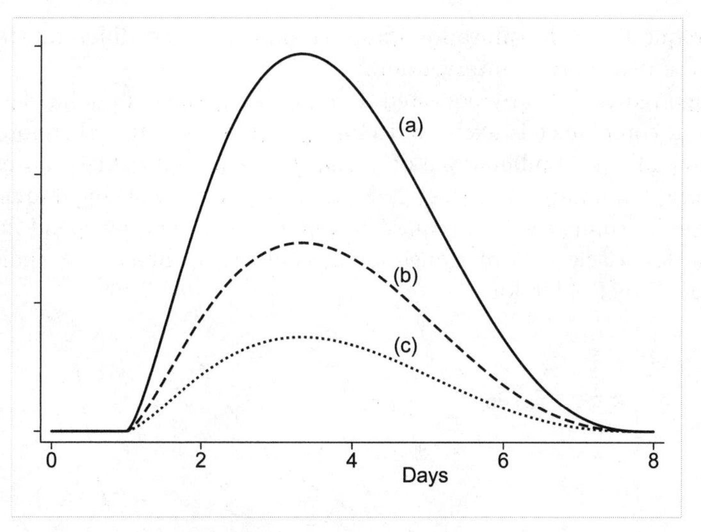

Figure 7.1 *Three illustrative transmission intensities between an infective-susceptible pair of individuals. In (a) neither the infective nor the susceptible have changed their mixing rate, i.e., both are non-responders. In (b) the infective is a person who halved his mixing rate and the susceptible mixes as usual. In (c) both the infective and the susceptible halved their mixing rate.*

where R_0 is the reproduction number when no one responds and $R_1 = a^2 R_0$ is the effective reproduction number when everyone responds. We can prevent an epidemic if every individual reduces their public mixing by a factor a provided a is small enough to make $R_1 = a^2 R_0 < 1$. That is, provided $a < 1/\sqrt{R_0}$. When this is so, the critical value for the fraction who comply is

$$f^{\dagger} = \frac{1 - 1/R_0}{1 - a^2}. \tag{7.2}$$

That is, a minor outbreak is certain when the fraction of individuals who are responders exceeds $f^{\dagger}$.

By comparing the type-specific mean matrices (6.2) and (7.1) we see that getting a fraction f of community members to reduce their mixing affects the mean matrix in the same way as vaccinating a fraction f of community members with a vaccine for which the susceptibility effect is a and the infectivity effects is also a. While the form of the effect is the same for these two control measures, the interpretation of each of the parameters a and f differs for the two types of intervention. The vaccine effect a has a biological basis, whereas the reduced mixing factor a has a social basis. The fraction f is the vaccination coverage when intervention is by vaccine, while for a request to reduce social mixing f is the fraction who comply with that request. Likely values for these parameters could differ substantially for these two types of intervention.

When individuals are requested to reduce their time in public places by a factor a, compliance is likely to decline as a decreases. It is therefore useful to know all the combinations of a and f values that achieve an effective reproduction number less than 1. A population survey asking individuals if they would comply with a request to reduce the time they spend in public places, for a selection of values for a, could then inform the choice of a suitable target value for a.

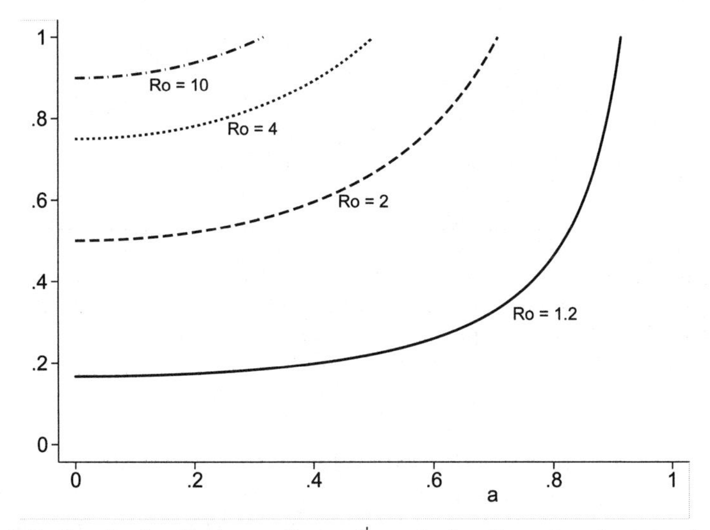

Figure 7.2 *Graph of critical compliance* $f^{\dagger}$ *against* a*, the reduced-mixing fraction, for four values of* R_0*.*

Figure 7.2 shows the graph of $f^{\dagger}$, as given by Equation (7.2), when R_0 takes values 1.2, 2, 4 and 10. For each R_0, values above the curve indicate points (a, f) for which the effective reproduction number is less than 1. Referring responses obtained in a compliance survey to this graph can help to determine which target value of a should be used in a request to reduce social mixing.

7.3 Isolating symptomatic infectives

It is natural for public health authorities to consider isolating infectives following diagnosis of their infection when looking for a strategy to control transmission of an infectious disease. Isolating infectives has the advantage of targeting only individuals who are actually infected. As such, public acceptance and compliance can be relatively high, particularly for an infectious disease with severe, or unknown, illness.

Isolation can sometimes play a major role in the control of an outbreak. For example, isolating symptomatic infectives played a major role in the control of Severe Acute Respiratory Syndrome (SARS) outbreaks, when SARS emerged in 2002. The key reason why isolating symptomatic infectives was effective is the fact that individuals infected with SARS become symptomatic close to the start of their infectious period. This characteristic of SARS enabled health authorities to reduce the time delay from onset of symptoms to isolation of the infective sufficiently to bring the effective reproduction number of SARS below 1.

7.3.1 How isolation changes the transmission intensity

To demonstrate how we can model the effect of isolating symptomatic infectives we consider an infection in a uniformly mixing community of size $n+1$, where n is large. Suppose some infected individuals react to onset of symptoms by continuing their regular activity, while others respond by isolating themselves until they are well. To model the different reactions we need to incorporate two types of individual, namely non-responder (Type 1) and responder (Type 2). Let $\psi_1(u) = \frac{1}{n}\psi_\Sigma(u)$ denote transmission intensity between a Type 1 infective and any given susceptible community member, where $\psi_\Sigma(u)$ is an aggregated transmission intensity function. A plausible transmission intensity between a Type 2 infective and any given susceptible is

$$\psi_2(u) = \begin{cases} c\,\psi_1(u), & \text{for } u_{\mathrm{S}} < u < u_{\mathrm{W}}, \\ \psi_1(u), & \text{otherwise,} \end{cases}$$

when onset of symptoms occurs u_{S} time units after infection and u_{W} is the duration from infection until the infective feels well again following his symptomatic period. Complete isolation is achieved during the symptomatic period when the constant $c = 0$.

If we take curve (a) in Figure 7.1 to be the transmission intensity $\psi_1(u)$, then Figure 7.3 illustrates two scenarios for the transmission intensity $\psi_2(u)$. According to curve (a) of Figure 7.3, the Type 2 infective mixes normally until the onset of symptoms, which occurs $u_{\mathrm{S}} = 2$ days after his infection. He then halves his mixing rate for three days, after which he becomes asymptomatic again and resumes his normal mixing rate. Curve (b) of Figure 7.3 illustrates a scenario in which an individual had reduced his mixing rate by 60% in response to an earlier public health request and upon becoming symptomatic he halved that mixing rate until the end of his infectious period.

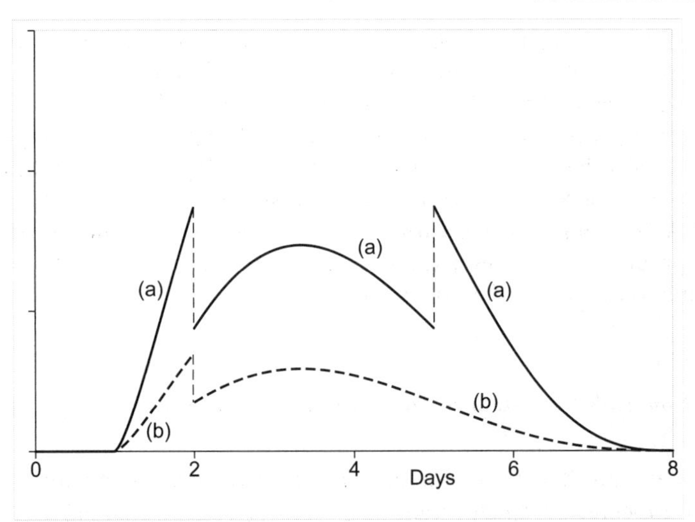

Figure 7.3 *Two illustrative transmission intensities between an infective-susceptible pair of individuals. In (a) the infective reduces his mixing rate while symptomatic, becoming asymptomatic again before the end of the infectious period. In (b) the infective is a person who reduced his mixing rate by 60% and, in addition, halves his mixing rate upon onset of symptoms.*

7.3.2 Impact on the reproduction number

We determine how a policy of isolating infectives upon onset of symptoms changes the reproduction number for two community settings.

A uniformly mixing community

The effect partial or complete isolation of symptomatic infectives has on the reproduction number is easily quantified for a community consisting of homogeneous susceptibles who mix uniformly. To illustrate, assume that a fraction f of infectives are totally isolated at onset of symptoms, which occurs $u_{\rm S}$ days after their infection, and the remaining infectives are not isolated. Following this public health intervention the matrix for the mean number of offspring generated by non-responding and responding infectives becomes

$$\begin{pmatrix} \mu_{11}^* & \mu_{12}^* \\ \mu_{21}^* & \mu_{22}^* \end{pmatrix} = \begin{pmatrix} \tilde{f}R_0 & fR_0 \\ b\tilde{f}R_0 & bfR_0 \end{pmatrix}, \tag{7.3}$$

where b is the fraction by which the total area under the transmission intensity function is reduced by the isolation. That is, $b =$(area under ψ_2)/(area under ψ_1). Comparing mean matrix (7.3) with the type-specific mean matrix (6.2), we deduce that the effect isolation of symptomatic infectives has on the mean matrix is of the same form as the effect when a fraction f of individuals are vaccinated with a vaccine that reduces infectivity only. However, again the interpretations of the parameters f and b differ in the two settings. In particular, parameter b in (6.2) has a biological basis, whereas in (7.3) the interpretation of b is based on a change in the rate of social mixing.

We deduce that the post-intervention reproduction number takes the familiar form $R^* = \tilde{f}R_0 + fR_1$, where R_0 is the basic reproduction number and, in this context, $R_1 = bR_0$ is the reproduction number when every infective is isolated at onset of symptoms.

Community of households

To illustrate the effect isolating symptomatic infectives has on the household reproduction number we consider a community consisting of a large number of households with each household comprised of two susceptibles. Suppose a fraction $\tilde{f}$ of households are of Type 1 and a fraction f are of Type 2. Members of Type 1 households are non-responders, meaning they are not isolated when infected and members of Type 2 households are responders, who are isolated at onset of symptoms. We assume that isolation is complete for each isolated infective, so that an infective is not able to infect anyone when isolated.

The household reproduction number is $R_{\text{H0}} = \mu(2 - q)$ when there is no isolation of infectives. To incorporate the effect of isolating a fraction f of symptomatic infectives we can proceed as for vaccinating a fraction f of community members with a vaccine that only reduces infectivity; see Section 6.2.2. We deduce that the effective household reproduction number becomes

$$R_{\text{H}} = \tilde{f}R_{\text{H0}} + fR_{\text{H1}},$$

where $R_{\text{H1}} = b\mu(2 - q^b)$ is the reproduction number when all symptomatic infectives are isolated.

7.4 Targeting high transmission intensities

Common sense suggests that the value of the reproduction number can be reduced effectively by focusing public health measures on any detected prominent sources of infection. For example, observing that case incidence is clustered in households suggests that interventions should target within-household transmission. On the other hand, observing that cases are disproportionately high for children suggests that a measure such as closing schools should be considered.

7.4.1 Quarantining infected households

The occurrence of multiple cases per infected household suggests that substantial potential for further transmission is generated within infected households. One way to mitigate the potential for infected households to reproduce is to immediately quarantine any household with a confirmed case of the infection. We now illustrate how to quantify the effect of quarantining infected households on the household reproduction number.

At the same time we take the opportunity to demonstrate an alternative way to model transmission in a community of households. Specifically, we introduce a way to model progression of the infection from household to household, taking "infected household" as the unit that reproduces.

For our setting we choose a community in which every household has two susceptibles and choose transmission intensity functions of a specific form. This is a conveniently simple setting in which to illustrate the essential features of modeling the effect of quarantining households.

Assumed form for the transmission intensity functions

We need to specify the transmission intensity acting between an infective-susceptible pair of individuals who are household partners and the transmission intensity acting between an infective-susceptible pair where the individuals are from different households. Each of these two transmission intensities is described by a function of the form

$$\psi(u) = \begin{cases} 0, & \text{for } 0 \le u \le u_{\text{L}}, \\ \beta, & \text{for } u_{\text{L}} < u < u_{\text{L}} + u_{\text{I}}, \\ 0 & \text{for } u \ge u_{\text{L}} + u_{\text{I}}, \end{cases}$$

where u_{L} is the duration of the latent period and u_{I} is the duration of the infectious period. The transmission coefficient β has two forms, depending on the type of infective-susceptible pair. It is given by

$$\beta = \begin{cases} \beta_{\text{H}}, & \text{for a pair of household partners,} \\ \frac{1}{n}\beta_{\text{C}}, & \text{for a pair of individuals from different households.} \end{cases}$$

With this specification the transmission intensity acting between a pair of individuals is constant over the infectious period, but the intensity may differ for within-household and between-household pairs.

A reproduction number for infected households

To model the reproduction of infected households we need to compute the mean number of infected households generated by a typical infected household. We do this by summing the mean number of households infected by each member of the infected household. Consider first the case when no public health intervention is in place.

The mean number of households infected by the primary household infective is $\beta_C u_I$. The number of households infected by the household partner of the primary infective has an additional element of chance. He infects zero households when he avoids infection by his household partner, but when he does become infected he also infects a mean of $\beta_C u_I$ households. The events of "avoiding infection" and "being infected" by the primary household infective occur with probability $\exp(-\beta_H u_I)$ and $1-\exp(-\beta_H u_I)$, respectively. We deduce that the mean number of households infected by the household partner of the primary infective is $\beta_C u_I[1-\exp(-\beta_H u_I)]$.

Adding the mean number of households infected by the primary infective and the mean number infected by his household partner gives the pre-intervention household reproduction number

$$R_{H0} = \beta_C u_I[2-\exp(-\beta_H u_I)].$$

This is seen to agree with the expression $R_H = \mu\nu_H$ given by (3.1), because in the present setting with the present notation $\mu = \beta_C u_I$ and the mean outbreak size in an infected household is $\nu_H = 2-\exp(-\beta_H u_I)$.

Our derivation shows that the household reproduction number based on the modified allocation of offspring to an infective, as described in Section 3.1, is the same as the reproduction number obtained by taking infected households as the units of infection.

The effect of quarantining on the household reproduction number

We now introduce quarantining of infected households. Assume each infective becomes symptomatic u_Q days after being infected and that $u_L \leq u_Q \leq u_L + u_I$. In other words, infectives become symptomatic during their infectious period. A household is quarantined when the primary household infective becomes symptomatic and we assume that infectives cannot infect anyone outside their household after their household is quarantined.

With this household quarantining measure in place the mean number of households the primary infective infects is $\beta_C(u_Q - u_L)$. To get the household reproduction number, we need to add to this the mean number of households infected by the household partner of the primary infective. Allowing for latent periods, we deduce that the household partner does not become infectious before quarantine time u_Q if $u_Q < 2u_L$. Therefore, quarantining households reduces the household reproduction number from $R_{H0} = \beta_C u_I[2-\exp(-\beta_H u_I)]$ to $R^*_{HQ} = \beta_C(u_Q - u_L)$ when $u_Q < 2u_L$.

Now suppose $u_Q > 2u_L$. The household partner of the primary infective can only infect other households if (i) he becomes infected, and (ii) his random infection time U falls into the period from u_L to $u_Q - u_L$ days following the infection of the primary household infective. Given that the household partner is infected and his infection time $U = u$, where $u_L \leq u \leq u_Q - u_L$, the mean number of households that the secondary household case infects is

$$\beta_C(u_Q - u_L - u).$$

In Section 7.7 we average this over the possible values of u.

In summary, we find the household reproduction number when infected households are quarantined u_Q days after being infected to be

$$R^*_{HQ} = \begin{cases} \beta_C(u_Q - u_L), & \text{if } u_Q \leq 2u_L, \\ \beta_C(2u_Q - 3u_L) - \frac{\beta_C}{\beta_H}\{1 - \exp[-\beta_H(u_Q - 2u_L)]\}, & \text{if } u_Q > 2u_L. \end{cases}$$

Quarantining infected households versus isolating symptomatic infectives

To illustrate the effect of quarantining infected households on the household reproduction number we consider a numerical example, using the above household setting. To add interest we compare its effect with the corresponding effect seen when, instead of quarantining households, we isolate every infective at onset of symptoms. It is clear that quarantining households will give the greater reduction in the household reproduction number, because, under quarantining, secondary household infectives tend to be prevented from infecting other households earlier. However, isolating infectives has the advantage of imposing only on infectives. Therefore quarantining households would only be justified if it is demonstrated to be substantially more effective than isolating symptomatic infectives.

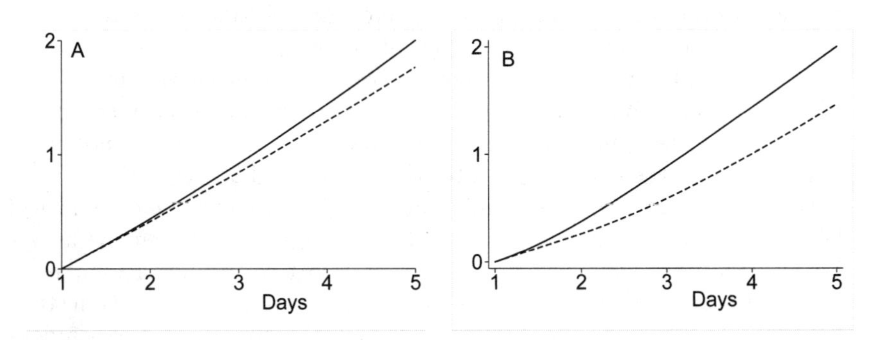

Figure 7.4 *Post-intervention household reproduction number when the intervention is (i) infectives are isolated at onset of symptoms (solid line), and (ii) infected households are quarantined at onset of symptoms in primary infective (dashed line). The basic reproduction number is $R_{H0} = 2$ in all four scenarios. The graphs in A compare the interventions when within-household transmission is modest and the graphs in B compare them when within-household transmission is high.*

As mentioned, the basic reproduction number in the above setting is $R_{\text{H0}} = \beta_{\text{C}} u_{\text{I}}[2 - \exp(-\beta_{\text{H}} u_{\text{I}})]$. The intervention of quarantining households reduces this to R^*_{HQ}, given above, and the intervention of isolating individuals at onset of symptoms has a post-intervention reproduction number

$$R^*_{\text{H}\mathcal{I}} = \beta_{\text{C}}(u_{\text{Q}} - u_{\text{L}})\{2 - \exp[-\beta_{\text{H}}(u_{\text{Q}} - u_{\text{L}})]\}.$$

In Figure 7.4 we compare these two post-intervention household reproduction numbers for two sets of parameters. In both scenarios we used a latent period of one day ($u_{\text{L}} = 1$), an infectious period of four days ($u_{\text{I}} = 4$) and $R_{\text{H0}} = 2$. Their difference lies in the rate of within-household transmission. The graphs in pane A of Figure 7.4 assume that the probability of the primary infective infecting his household partner is $1 - \exp(-4\beta_{\text{H}}) = 0.2$ and for the graphs in pane B of Figure 7.4 this probability is 0.9. In each case the value of β_{C} is chosen to make $R_{\text{H0}} = 2$. The graphs in Figure 7.4 illustrate that quarantining infected households is able to produce an effective reproduction number that is lower than that produced by isolating infectives at onset of symptoms, but the difference is modest unless the within-household transmission rate is high. A different conclusion can be reached when households are larger.

7.4.2 Social distancing of a type of individual

Sometimes a specific group of individuals is identified as a major source of spread of the infection and there is interest in focusing social distancing interventions on this group. To illustrate, assume that children play a larger role in spreading a certain infection than adults. The difference in the transmission rate may be biological or social. For example, children may have a less developed immune system and therefore are more susceptible and be infectious for a longer period of time. Alternatively, the social habits of children, including attendance at school, may be the source of this difference. We briefly explore these two scenarios, without including a household structure.

Individuals differ biologically

First consider a biological explanation for the difference in the susceptibility and infectivity of adults (Type 1) and children (Type 2). A reasonable way to model this difference is to proceed as we did for unvaccinated and vaccinated individuals. That is, much like in Equation (6.2), we propose a type-specific mean matrix of the form

$$\begin{pmatrix} \mu_{11} & \mu_{12} \\ \mu_{21} & \mu_{22} \end{pmatrix} = \begin{pmatrix} f_1\mu & af_2\mu \\ bf_1\mu & abf_2\mu \end{pmatrix},$$

where f_1 is the fraction of individuals that is adults and $f_2 = 1 - f_1$ is the fraction that is children. In contrast to the vaccination setting, we might now have a and b greater than 1, which means that children are more effective conduits of the infection.

As a step towards assessing social distancing interventions, suppose it is possible to get all children to reduce their mixing to a fraction c of their normal mixing rate. The mean matrix would then become

$$\begin{pmatrix} f_1\mu & acf_2\mu \\ bcf_1\mu & abc^2 f_2\mu \end{pmatrix}.$$

This intervention reduces the reproduction number from $R = f_1\mu + abf_2\mu$ to $R^* = f_1\mu + abc^2 f_2\mu$.

Social mixing differs between individuals

Suppose now that the difference in the transmission rate is due to a difference in mixing rates. It could be that the number of individuals contacted differs or the proportion of close contacts differs. Suppose, for example, that the difference in the transmission rate is primarily explained by the close and constant contact children have with each other at school. We outline a simple way to quantify the effect of closing schools on transmission of the infectious disease.

Divide each day into three parts: 8 hours of sleep, when no transmission of the infection occurs, 8 hours of "school time" and the remaining 8 hours when general "community mixing" takes place.

The part of the initial mean matrix corresponding to the community-mixing time segment might be described by

$$\begin{pmatrix} f_1\mu & f_2\mu \\ f_1\mu & f_2\mu \end{pmatrix},$$

where $f_2 = 1 - f_1$ is the fraction of individuals that is schoolchildren. This mean matrix corresponds to uniform mixing, so that close contacts by infectives with adults and children occur according to their relative abundance in the community.

The part of the mean matrix corresponding to the school time segment might be described by

$$\begin{pmatrix} af_1\mu & 0 \\ 0 & bf_2\mu \end{pmatrix},$$

where a reflects the change in the rate of close mixing among adults when children are at school and b reflects the change in the rate of close mixing among children when they are at school. The zeros in this component of the mean matrix indicate that during school time there is minimal cross-mixing between adults and schoolchildren.

Adding these two mean matrices gives the overall mean matrix

$$\begin{pmatrix} \mu_{11} & \mu_{12} \\ \mu_{21} & \mu_{22} \end{pmatrix} = \begin{pmatrix} (1+a)f_1\mu & f_2\mu \\ f_1\mu & (1+b)f_2\mu \end{pmatrix}.$$

Substituting the elements of this mean matrix into Equation (4.2) gives the reproduction number

$$R = \frac{\mu}{2}\left(1 + af_1 + bf_2 + \sqrt{(f_1 + af_1 - f_2 - bf_2)^2 + 4f_1 f_2}\right).$$

When schools are closed the mean matrix for school time is plausibly the same as the mean matrix for community-mixing time and the overall mean matrix becomes

$$\begin{pmatrix} \mu_{11}^* & \mu_{12}^* \\ \mu_{21}^* & \mu_{22}^* \end{pmatrix} = \begin{pmatrix} 2f_1\mu & 2f_2\mu \\ 2f_1\mu & 2f_2\mu \end{pmatrix},$$

for which the corresponding reproduction number is $R^* = 2\mu$. As a consequence, it is possible to bring the reproduction number below 1 by closing schools if $\mu < \frac{1}{2}$.

As always, when drawing conclusions it is important to be aware of the assumptions made in the model. For example, the assumptions made here are not appropriate if closing schools means that schoolchildren use the usual school time to play with each other elsewhere rather than engaging in general community mixing.

7.5 Discussion

Social distancing measures to mitigate transmission of an infectious disease play a major part in preparedness plans for emerging infectious diseases. For example, when human swine influenza emerged in 2009 a disproportionate number of children were diagnosed with the disease and in some affected locations schools were closed as part of their pandemic outbreak response. It turned out that the 2009 outbreak of human swine influenza was well suited to interventions that focus on children, because in many affected regions the mean number infected per child infective was greater than 1 and the mean number infected per adult infective was a little below 1.

Social distancing measures are also finding applications in the control of infectious disease that circulate regularly. For example, ill-founded information about side effects of the vaccine has led some parents not to vaccinate their children against measles, with the consequence that, in some regions, the immunity coverage has become inadequate and the effective reproduction number has increased to a value above 1. This means that outbreaks are possible and some schools have been given the authority to send unvaccinated pupils home for the duration of a school outbreak of measles.

7.6 Exercises

1. Of the individuals in a large community a proportion f_1 are of Type 1 and a proportion $f_2 = 1 - f_1$ are of Type 2. These types of individual differ only in that Type 2 individuals regularly attend mass gathering events, such as popular sporting events and concerts. To protect against the risk that the introduction of a newly emerged infection leads to an epidemic, the community's health service is studying how much a ban on mass gathering events would reduce the value of the effective reproduction number when such an infection is introduced.

   Suppose the mean number of infectives generated by Type 1 and Type 2 individuals during the initial stage of an outbreak is given by

$$\begin{pmatrix} \mu_{11} & \mu_{12} \\ \mu_{21} & \mu_{22} \end{pmatrix} = \begin{pmatrix} f_1\mu & f_2\mu \\ f_1\mu & f_2\mu + a\mu \end{pmatrix}$$

   where the term $a\mu$ reflects the mean number of infections a Type 2 infective generates at mass gathering events.

   (a) Find an expression for R_{T}, the reproduction number associated with this type-specific mean matrix.

   (b) Let R_{T}^* denote the reproduction number when a complete ban on mass gathering events is imposed.

   On the same graph sketch the curves of $R_{\mathrm{T}}^*/R_{\mathrm{T}}$ against a when (i) $f_1 = 0.1$ and (ii) $f_1 = 0.9$.

   What do these curves tell us about the effectiveness of banning mass gathering events?

2. A new infectious disease has emerged. Suppose the reproduction number of this infectious disease is R_0 in a large uniformly mixing community that has not yet had any cases. Their public health authority issues a request for people to reduce their rate of mixing.

   (a) Find an expression for the reproduction number if 40% of individuals reduce their public interaction to 50% of their usual mixing rate and the other 60% of individuals do not change their mixing rate.

   What is the largest value of R_0 for which this level of compliance with the public health request will prevent an epidemic?

   (b) Find the reproduction number if 70% of individuals reduce their public interaction to 80% of their usual mixing rate and the remaining 30% reduce their mixing in public to 20% of their usual mixing rate.

   What is the largest value of R_0 for which this level reduced mixing will prevent an epidemic?

3. Consider a community of $n + 1$ homogeneous individuals who mix uniformly, where n is large. All are susceptible to a certain infectious disease.

The transmission intensity between a primary infective of this infectious disease and a given susceptible is $\frac{1}{n}\psi(u)$, where

$$\psi(u) = \begin{cases} 0, & \text{if } 0 \le u < 1, \\ 4(u-1), & \text{if } 1 \le u < 2, \\ 2(4-u), & \text{if } 2 \le u < 4, \\ 0, & \text{if } u \ge 4. \end{cases}$$

All infectives have a two day symptomatic period, which begins exactly 1.5 days after the time of their infection.

Two public health interventions are being considered for the control of outbreaks of this infectious disease.

`Intervention A`: All infectives are isolated while they are symptomatic.

`Intervention B`: A fraction f of individuals, independently, reduce their mixing rate by 50%. (Others mix as usual.)

Let R_0 denote the basic reproduction number and let $R_{\mathtt{A}}^*$ and $R_{\mathtt{B}}^*$ be the initial reproduction numbers under interventions A and B, respectively.

Find the value of

(a) R_0,
(b) $R_{\mathtt{A}}^*$ and
(c) the minimum value of f such that $R_{\mathtt{B}}^* \le R_{\mathtt{A}}^*$.

4. A large community consists of households of size two, with both members susceptible to a newly emerged infectious disease. The basic household reproduction number is $R_{\text{H0}} = \mu\nu_{\text{H}}$, where μ is the mean number of households an infective infects and ν_{H} is the mean outbreak size in an infected household.

From disease transmission observed elsewhere, public health officers know that infection occurs only during close contact, defined as "interaction between individuals who are less than 1 m apart."

Consider an intervention consisting of an official request that people reduce the number of close contacts they have in public places. In response, 50% of all individuals reduce the number of close contacts they have in public places to $100a$% of their usual mixing in public. The other 50% of individuals make no change to their public mixing.

(a) Find an expression for R_{HA}^*, the post-intervention initial reproduction number when the responders consist of both members of one-half of the households.
Determine the range of values for a that prevent an epidemic if $R_{\text{H0}} = 1.6$.

(b) Find an expression for R^*_{HB}, the post-intervention initial reproduction number when the responders consist of one member from every household.

(c) Find an expression for reproduction numbers R^*_{HA} and R^*_{HB} when $a = 0.6$ and $\nu_{\text{H}} = 1.9$.

Compare their values.

(d) Show that $R^*_{\text{HB}} \leq R^*_{\text{HA}}$ for all values of the parameters a, μ and ν_{H}.

5. A community with a large adult population is currently free from a certain sexually transmissible disease (STD) and is considering strategies to minimize the chance that an introduction of the infection will lead to an epidemic. Assume that the probability of transmission to a sexual partner is not dependent on who is the infective and who is the susceptible.

Eighty percent of sexually active adults live with a partner and the remaining 20% of sexually active adults are single. Ninety percent of couples consist of partners that are faithful. That is, they have sex only with their partner. Every individual in the other 10% of couples, occasionally, independently and randomly, has sex with a single individual. Single individuals have multiple single sex partners and occasionally have sex with an individual from a couple.

It is estimated, from a survey of sexual activity, that a single infective would infect an average of 3.5 single individuals and 0.2 individuals from a couple during the early stage of an outbreak of this STD. An infective from one of the promiscuous couples is estimated to infect their partner with probability 0.4 and an average of 0.1 single individuals.

(a) By treating an infected single individual as an outbreak in a household of size one and an infected couple as an outbreak in a household of size two, or otherwise, compute a basic reproduction number for the STD in this community.

(b) Assuming that use of a condom during sex provides full protection against this STD, what proportion of the single individuals needs to use a condom during all sex to ensure epidemics of this STD are prevented?

(c) Explain why use of condoms can be viewed as a social distancing intervention.

7.7 Supplementary material

Household reproduction number when infected households are quarantined

Consider a large community consisting of households with two susceptible members, as in Section 7.4.1. To derive the expression for the household reproduction number under quarantining, we need to sum over the mean number of households infected by each member of an infected household. Using the notation of Section 7.4.1, the primary household infective infects a mean number of $\beta_{\mathrm{C}}(u_{\mathrm{Q}} - u_{\mathrm{L}})$ households. His household partner can infect other households only if he is infected by the primary household infective *and* he becomes infectious before the household is quarantined. Suppose that the primary household infective infects his household partner U days after his own infection, where U is random. Then conditionally, given $U = u$, the mean number of households infected by the secondary household infective is

$$g(u) = \begin{cases} \beta_{\mathrm{C}}(u_{\mathrm{Q}} - u_{\mathrm{L}} - u), & \text{if } u_{\mathrm{L}} \leq u \leq u_{\mathrm{Q}} - u_{\mathrm{L}}, \\ 0, & \text{if } u > u_{\mathrm{Q}} - u_{\mathrm{L}}. \end{cases}$$

Unconditionally, the mean number of households infected by the secondary household infective is

$$\begin{aligned} \mathrm{E}[g(U)] &= \beta_{\mathrm{C}} \int_{u_{\mathrm{L}}}^{u_{\mathrm{Q}} - u_{\mathrm{L}}} (u_{\mathrm{Q}} - u_{\mathrm{L}} - u)\beta_{\mathrm{H}} \exp[-\beta_{\mathrm{H}}(u - u_{\mathrm{L}})]\, du \\ &= \beta_{\mathrm{C}}(u_{\mathrm{Q}} - 2u_{\mathrm{L}}) - \frac{\beta_{\mathrm{C}}}{\beta_{\mathrm{H}}}\{1 - \exp[-\beta_{\mathrm{H}}(u_{\mathrm{Q}} - 2u_{\mathrm{L}})]\}. \end{aligned}$$

Adding the mean number of households infected by the primary infective and the mean number infected by his household partner we find the household reproduction number when infected households are quarantined u_{Q} days after being infected to be

$$R^*_{\mathrm{HQ}} = \beta_{\mathrm{C}}(2u_{\mathrm{Q}} - 3u_{\mathrm{L}}) - \frac{\beta_{\mathrm{C}}}{\beta_{\mathrm{H}}}\{1 - \exp[-\beta_{\mathrm{H}}(u_{\mathrm{Q}} - 2u_{\mathrm{L}})]\}.$$

7.8 Bibliographic notes

Caley et al. (2008) use modeling to find evidence that social distancing is likely to have occurred during the 1918–1919 influenza pandemic. Glass and Barnes (2007) and Cauchemez et al. (2008) find evidence that school closure is likely to reduce the transmission of influenza. Cauchemez et al. (2009) review the multiple aspects of school closure as a public health policy.

The papers by Ferguson et al. (2006) and Glass et al. (2006) demonstrate how modeling can be used to assess the likely impact of social distancing measures and to design effective strategies to mitigate the impact of pandemic influenza.

CHAPTER 8

Reducing epidemic size

Consider a large community that is currently free from a certain infectious disease, for which the effective reproduction number R is greater than 1. Figure 2.6 illustrates that importation of the infection has two distinct types of outcome when $R > 1$. Either a minor outbreak occurs or an epidemic. Which of these outcomes occurs is subject to chance. Specifically, it depends on whether the number of infectives builds up adequately during the early stage of the outbreak for transmission "to take off."

Previous chapters discuss minor outbreaks, including the probability that an outbreak will be minor and the size of minor outbreaks. The size of minor outbreaks that occur when $R > 1$ has also been touched upon. We now add discussion on the other possible outcome when $R > 1$, namely the epidemic.

When assessing measures aimed at controlling outbreaks initiated by *occasional introductions* of the infection, it is important to consider both the chance that the outbreak will become an epidemic and the size of a potential epidemic. In contrast, when there are *multiple introductions* it is almost certain that an epidemic will occur, when $R > 1$, and control planning can then focus primarily on ways to reduce the size of the epidemic. Both types of introduction of the infection are helped by having a way to study the effect of public health interventions on the eventual size of an epidemic that might occur.

Unless stated otherwise, this chapter assumes that the initial reproduction number is larger than 1.

8.1 Simulated epidemics

A useful first step is to see what simulated epidemics for different parameter values can tell us. Consider a community of 10,000 susceptible individuals who are homogeneous and mix uniformly. To simulate epidemics in this community we first fix a value for R, the initial reproduction number. To capture the element of chance, we then simulate 2000 outbreaks assuming that each outbreak is initiated by a single, newly infected individual and that the offspring distribution is Poisson. The mean number of offspring is R for the initial infective. To allow for the depletion of susceptibles we set the mean of the offspring distribution for each infective of generation j to be $R(1 - C_j/10000)$, where C_j is the total number of cases that occurred in previous generations of that epidemic. This allows for the depletion of susceptibles as the outbreak progresses.

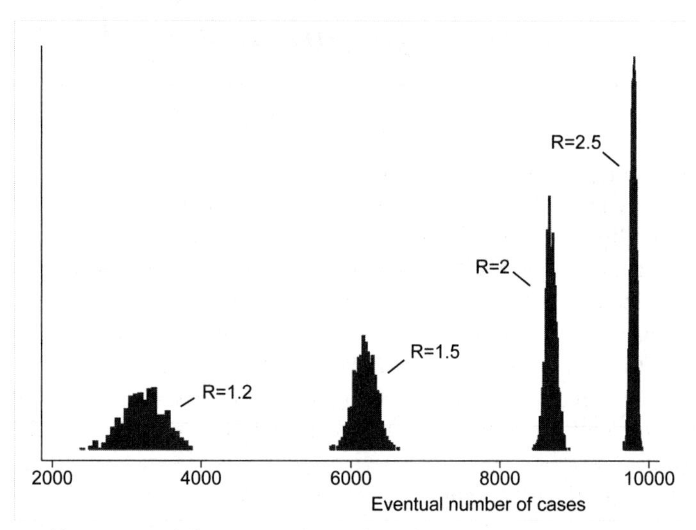

Figure 8.1 *Histogram of the eventual number of cases in 2000 simulated outbreaks, for each of four values of the initial reproduction number R. Cases for minor outbreaks are not shown. Each community initially had 10,000 susceptibles.*

Figure 8.1 shows the histogram of epidemic size for each of four sets of 2000 simulations. The values of the initial reproduction number, R, used in these simulations were 1.2, 1.5, 2.0 and 2.5, respectively. Each set of simulations included some minor outbreaks. These are not shown in Figure 8.1.

An immediate observation from these histograms is that epidemic sizes for each chosen R value are quite closely clustered around a central value. Clustering is tighter for larger values of R.

A second observation is that the central value for the total number of cases increases as R increases. This suggests that any public health intervention able to reduce the value of the initial reproduction number can reduce the eventual number of cases substantially. More broadly, it suggests that R plays a useful role in guiding public health management of epidemic size.

Figure 8.1 also shows that the eventual number of cases does not depend linearly on the value of R. It is therefore important to study the nature of this relationship if we want to use R to guide strategies for the control of infectious diseases.

Unfortunately the algebra of stochastic epidemic models for a large population is difficult, to the extent that computation runs into problems of numerical accuracy. This leads investigators to study the size of epidemics with the aid of computer simulations or by turning to deterministic models. We prefer, and adopt, the deterministic modeling approach because it is less laborious and, in our setting, leads to explicit formulae that are well suited to exploring the effectiveness of interventions.

8.2 The nature of our deterministic epidemic model

Deterministic models ignore the chance component in transmission. Chance is an important component while the number of infectives or susceptibles is small, but less so when describing the size of an epidemic in a large population. We get a glimpse of this in Figure 8.1, which shows that epidemic sizes are quite closely clustered. Clustering in the fraction infected in an epidemic is even tighter for larger populations. From a public health perspective the main interest lies in how the central epidemic size changes as R changes, and a deterministic model captures this aspect conveniently.

Let t denote the time elapsed since the infection was introduced into the community. An infectious disease model keeps track of $N(t)$, the number of individuals who have been infected by time t, and $S(t)$, the number of susceptibles remaining at time t. In practice $N(t)$ and $S(t)$ take only integer values. However, our deterministic model allows $N(t)$ and $S(t)$ to change by arbitrarily small amounts. In other words, $N(t)$ and $S(t)$ can take any value from 0 to the total size of the community. For such a model to be reasonable we need $N(t)$ and $S(t)$ to take large values, so that a change of one unit in either $N(t)$ or $S(t)$ is small relative to their values. During an epidemic in a large community this will be the case most of the time.

A considerable advantage of using a deterministic model is that it gives a single value for the size of an epidemic and an explicit formula can be obtained for this size. This makes a deterministic model a convenient tool for assessing the merits of different measures proposed for the management of epidemics.

Note that we use a deterministic description only for outbreaks that progress to become epidemics.

8.3 Epidemic size in a homogeneous community

Consider a large community of individuals who mix uniformly. Suppose a fraction s_0 of individuals is susceptible to an infectious disease that has a basic reproduction number R_0 in this community. We describe the epidemic size by y, the fraction of community members eventually infected when an epidemic occurs following the introduction of the infection by an external contact. The final-size equation,

$$s_0 - y = s_0 \exp(-R_0 y), \qquad (8.1)$$

is derived in Section 8.10.1. It can be solved, numerically, to give y for any specified values of s_0 and R_0.

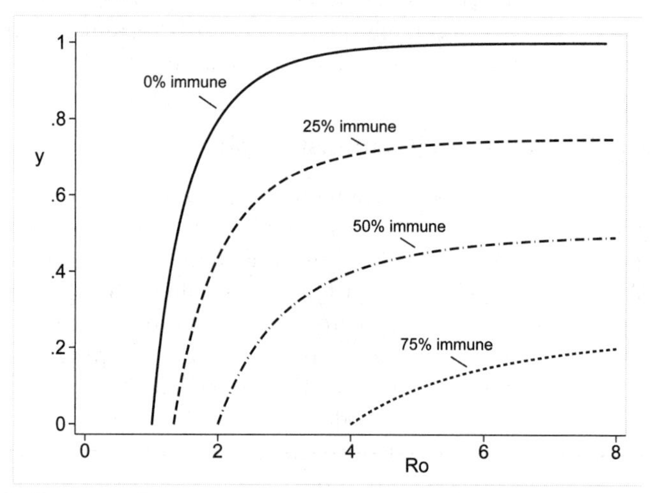

Figure 8.2 *Fraction of community members eventually infected for an infectious disease with basic reproduction number R_0, when the fraction of immune community members at the start of the outbreak is 0, 0.25, 0.5 and 0.75.*

The graphs in Figure 8.2 show how the community attack rate y increases as the value of R_0 increases, for situations with $s_0 = 1$, 0.75, 0.5 or 0.25. The solid curve gives the relationship between y and R_0 for a community with everyone susceptible and the lower three curves show how the attack rate is reduced when a fraction of the community members is immune at the start of the outbreak. Immunity at the start of the outbreak might be due to a combination of prior exposure and prior vaccination.

Two interesting observations can be made from the graphs in Figure 8.2. First, the solid graph shows that in a fully susceptible community virtually everyone is infected when R_0 is large, greater than 4 say. We should therefore expect this to happen for measles, which is thought to have an R_0 value greater than 15 in most communities. The epidemic data in Table 10.14 illustrate that this is indeed what is observed in practice.

Second, the attack rate is positive only for values of $R_0 > 1/s_0$. This fits well with the transmission threshold property stated on page 8, namely that epidemics are prevented when $R = s_0R_0$, the reproduction number at the start of the outbreak, is less than 1. In other words, on this point the deterministic model reaches a conclusion that is analogous to the one deduced from the stochastic model formulation. This agreement is always true for our deterministic model, not just for the four curves shown in Figure 8.2; see Section 8.10.2.

The deterministic final-size equation (8.1) provides no information about the size of minor outbreaks. The observation that $y = 0$ at $R_0 = 1/s_0$ means that this deterministic model, which assumes a large community, describes the eventual number of cases in a minor outbreak as negligible relative to the size of the population.

We now describe how the deterministic final-size equation (8.1), together with consideration of the chance elements associated with the introduction of an infection, can be used to quantify the effect of mass immunization on the attack rate.

8.4 Mass immunization

Consider a community that is currently free from a certain infectious disease. Conducting a mass immunization campaign against this infection protects community members in four ways:

(i) it lowers the eventual attack rate in the event of an epidemic,
(ii) it reduces the probability that an introduction of the infectious disease leads to an epidemic,
(iii) it reduces the probability that a contact by a community member with an external infective leads to an introduction of the infection, and
(iv) it bestows some protection against infection to community members who, for some reason, are unable to be immunized.

In this section we look at the first three of these effects of mass immunization. The fourth of the above features of mass immunization is discussed in the next section, under the heading of herd immunity.

Our setting is a large community consisting of homogeneous individuals who mix uniformly. We assume that a mass immunization campaign conducted in this community achieves vaccination coverage v, with a fully protective vaccine, and all unvaccinated individuals are fully susceptible to the infection. To see how effectively mass immunization mitigates transmission of the infectious disease we begin with a value of R_0 and look at the extent to which the community attack rate is reduced as the vaccination coverage v is increased.

8.4.1 Attack rate, given that an epidemic occurs

The effect of mass immunization on the expected attack rate when an epidemic occurs is sometimes of particular interest. For example, we might be concerned about the impact of an epidemic on the labor force or the burden of hospitalizations from the infectious disease during an epidemic.

In the event of an epidemic, the effect mass immunization has on the community attack rate is reflected implicitly in the graphs of Figure 8.2. However, a graph obtained by fixing the value of R_0 and then plotting the community attack rate y against the prior level of immunity $v = 1 - s_0$ shows the effect of mass immunization more directly.

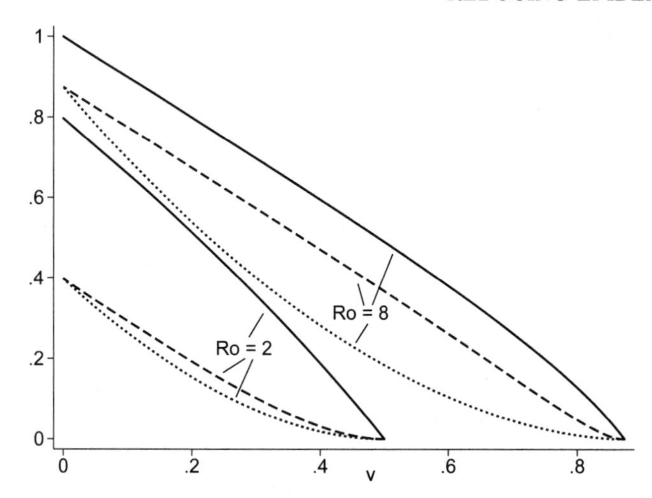

Figure 8.3 *Fraction of community members eventually infected for an infectious disease with basic reproduction number R_0 equal to 2 or 8, as the fraction of immunized community members varies.*
Solid curves show the attack rate given that an epidemic occurs.
Dashed curves include the possibility that the outbreak might be minor.
Dotted curves include the further possibility that a contact with an external infective might not lead to an introduction of the infectious disease.

For each of the values 2 and 8 for R_0, Figure 8.3 shows three graphs that display the expected eventual attack rate as v changes. The solid curves show the eventual attack rate y given that an epidemic occurs, from which we make two observations that have control implications:

(i) the attack rate y becomes zero before everyone is immunized, and
(ii) y decreases as v increases, with a gradient less than -1 at every point, for each of the two solid curves.

The first observation is not new. It shows that the deterministic model reflects the transmission threshold property of Section 2.1. The second observation gives a new insight, namely that each additional vaccine administered decreases the community attack rate by more than one case. In Section 8.10.3 this observation is generalized and made more precise. It is found that the number of cases by which the community attack rate is decreased (per vaccine administered) increases as the effective reproduction number R decreases, reaching two cases prevented per vaccine administered as R approaches 1.

8.4.2 Attack rate, given that an infection is introduced

When the initial reproduction number is greater than 1, the deterministic equation (8.1) gives the eventual attack rate in the event of an epidemic.

The deterministic model does not acknowledge the chance that an epidemic may not occur when the infection is introduced into the community. This is acceptable when there are multiple introductions, because then the chance of an epidemic is high. However, it is appropriate to acknowledge the chance of a minor outbreak when there are only occasional introductions of the infection.

For this discussion we take the eventual proportion of community members infected as 0 when an introduced infection leads to a minor outbreak. This approximation is based on the fact that the total number of cases in a minor outbreak is very small when compared to the number of cases in the event of an epidemic in this large community. With this approximation the weighted average of the attack rate, when the infection is introduced by one newly infected individual, is

$$\mathrm{av}_1(y) \;=\; 0 \times \pi \;+\; y \times (1-\pi) \;=\; (1-\pi)y,$$

where π is the probability of a minor outbreak and y, the community attack rate when an epidemic occurs, is given by (8.1).

Allowing for the chance of a minor outbreak attributes a greater benefit to mass immunization because immunization also decreases $1-\pi$, the probability that an introduction by a single initial infective leads to an epidemic.

To illustrate the size of the change in $\mathrm{av}_1(y)$ we make a specific calculation assuming a geometric offspring distribution. The probability of a minor outbreak is then $1-\pi = 1-1/R = 1-1/[(1-v)R_0]$; see Equation (2.11). The two dashed curves in Figure 8.3 show the mean, or average, attack rate $\mathrm{av}_1(y)$ when the outbreak is initiated by a single introductory infective. Comparing the rate of decline in each dashed curve with the decline in the corresponding solid curve shows that, in situations where introductions of the infection are occasional, the benefit of a moderate immunization coverage is understated when we look only at its effect on the epidemic attack rate y.

8.4.3 Attack rate, given a close contact with an external infective

Mass immunization also reduces the probability that a contact between a community member and an external infective leads to an introduction of the infectious disease. A close contact between a community member and an external infective only introduces the infection when the community member is unvaccinated. Therefore the mean attack rate resulting from a single close contact between a randomly selected community member and an external infective is

$$\mathrm{av}_2(y) \;=\; (1-v)(1-\pi)y.$$

The two dotted curves in Figure 8.3 are the graphs of $\mathrm{av}_2(y)$ against v, the fraction of community members that is vaccinated, assuming a geometric offspring distribution. We see that this leads to an additional reduction in the mean attack rate. This reduction is appreciable for larger values of R_0.

8.5 Herd immunity

We now look at the benefit of mass immunization from a different angle, motivated by the fourth in the list of benefits of mass immunization given on page 125.

The term *herd immunity* is often used in infectious disease epidemiology, albeit with some variety in its definition. At the heart of each definition is the observation that susceptible community members who are not immunized acquire indirect protection against infection when some of their fellow community members are immunized. This observation is reflected in the curves of Figure 8.3, where both scenarios ($R_0 = 2$ and $R_0 = 8$) indicate that a community attack rate of zero can be achieved without immunizing everyone. In the following we suggest ways to quantify how much protection an unvaccinated individual acquires when some fellow community members are immunized.

Our setting is a large community consisting of homogeneous susceptibles who mix uniformly. A mass immunization campaign, with a fully protective vaccine, is conducted and achieves vaccination coverage v. For three different scenarios, each of which is specified by a realized event, we quantify the benefit an unvaccinated individual acquires from the immunization campaign. The three events are the same as those used in the previous section, namely:
Event 1: an epidemic occurs,
Event 2: the infection is introduced by one newly infected individual, and
Event 3: a community member has close contact with an external infective.

For $j = 1, 2$ and 3, we compute $p_j(v)$, the conditional probability that a specific unvaccinated individual is infected, given that Event j has occurred. The benefit an unvaccinated individual acquires from the immunization campaign is evident from a comparison of $p_j(v)$ with $p_j(0)$. Here $p_j(0)$ is the conditional probability that a specific unvaccinated individual is infected in a community with no one vaccinated, given that Event j has occurred.

8.5.1 An epidemic occurs

Given that an epidemic occurs, the probability that a specific susceptible is amongst those infected during the course of the epidemic is

$$p_1(v) \;=\; y_{\mathrm{S}} = y/s_0,$$

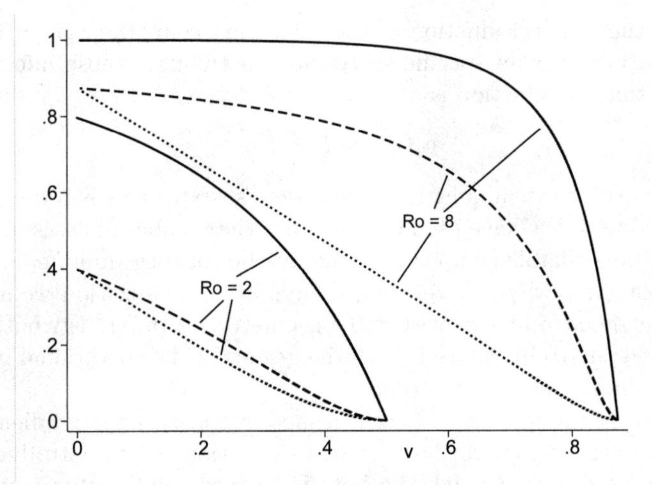

Figure 8.4 *Expected fraction of susceptible individuals infected for different values of v, the fraction of immunized community members.*
Solid curves show the expected fraction given that an epidemic occurs.
Dashed curves include the possibility that an outbreak might be minor.
Dotted curves include the further possibility that a contact with an external infective might not lead to an introduction of the infectious disease.

the attack rate among those who were susceptible at the start of the epidemic. From the deterministic final-size equation (8.1), with $s_0 = 1 - v$, we find

$$1 - y_{\mathrm{S}} \;=\; \exp[-R_0(1 - v)y_{\mathrm{S}}].$$

This equation can be solved for y_{S} when the value of $R_0(1 - v)$ is specified.

The solid curves in Figure 8.4 illustrate how $p_1(v) = y_{\mathrm{S}}$ decreases as v increases when R_0 has values 2 and 8. The intercept of each solid curve with the vertical axis shows that the probability of a given susceptible being infected is less than 1 even when there is no immunity, although the probability is close to 1 when R_0 has a large value, such as 8. The probability of being infected decreases as v increases, at a rate that depends on the value of R_0. As v approaches the critical immunity coverage, $p_1(v)$ decreases at its fastest rate, namely $2R_0$ (derived in Section 8.10.4). This is noteworthy for infectious disease control, because it tells us that an increase in the vaccination coverage has the greatest impact when the coverage v is close to its critical value.

8.5.2 The infectious disease is introduced

When introductions of the infection are occasional, a susceptible gains further protection against infection because the immunization campaign also decreases $1 - \pi$, the probability that an introduction leads to an epidemic.

Given that an introduction of the infection occurs, i.e., given Event 2, the probability that a specific susceptible is amongst those infected as a result of this introduction is

$$p_2(v) = (1-\pi)y_S,$$

the mean attack rate among those who were susceptible when the infection was introduced. We have used the fact that the number of cases in a minor outbreak is negligible compared to the number of cases in an epidemic.

To illustrate how $p_2(v)$ is changed by mass immunization we again assume a single introductory case and a geometric offspring distribution. The two dashed curves in Figure 8.4 are the graphs of the conditional probability $p_2(v)$ under these assumptions.

Comparing the gradient in each dashed curve with the gradient in the corresponding solid curve shows that, in situations where introductions of the infection are occasional, the benefit to susceptibles from a moderate immunization coverage is understated when we look only at its effect on $p_1(v)$, the attack rate among susceptibles in the event of an epidemic.

8.5.3 A community member contacts an external infective

When contacts with external infectives are occasional, a susceptible gains yet another component of protection against infection because the immunization campaign also increases the probability that a contact with an external infective fails to lead to an introduction.

A close contact between a randomly selected community member and an external infective only introduces the infection when the community member is unvaccinated. Therefore, given only that there is a close contact between a randomly selected community member and an external infective, i.e., given Event 3, the probability of a specific susceptible acquiring an infection during possible subsequent transmission is

$$p_3(v) = (1-v)(1-\pi)y_S.$$

The two dotted curves in Figure 8.3 are the graphs of $p_3(v)$ against v, the fraction of community members that is vaccinated. We see that the additional reduction in the probability that a susceptible is infected can be appreciable for larger values of R_0.

8.6 Estimating the reproduction number

The methods for estimating a reproduction number introduced in Sections 2.7 and 3.6 are based on incidence counts in the first few generations of an epidemic and on final-size counts from a number of minor outbreaks. We now assume that the overall attack rate in one entire epidemic is observed.

Our target is R, the initial reproduction number. Estimating its value will inform future planning for the management of this infectious disease.

To obtain an estimating equation we rewrite Equation (8.1) in the form

$$R = \frac{-\ln(1 - y_{\mathrm{S}})}{y_{\mathrm{S}}}, \tag{8.2}$$

where $R = R_0 s_0$ is the effective reproduction number at the start of the epidemic and $y_{\mathrm{S}} = y/s_0$ is the fraction of individuals infected during the epidemic among those susceptible at the start of the epidemic. This provides a way to estimate R when y_{S} is observed.

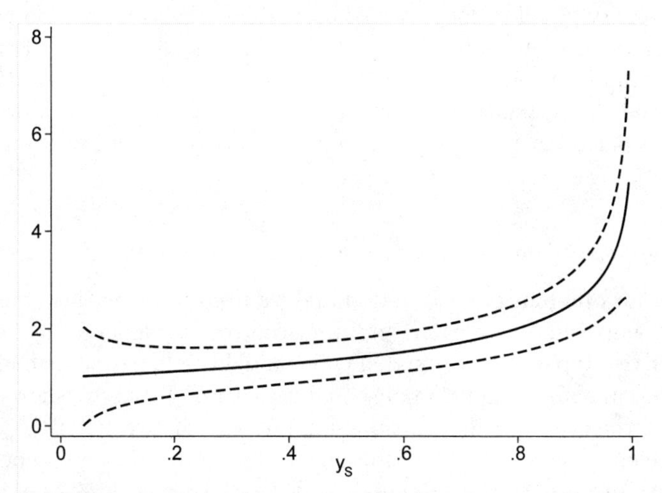

Figure 8.5 *Solid curve: estimate $\widehat{R}$ of R, the reproduction number at the start of the epidemic, corresponding to observation y_{S}, the fraction of community members eventually infected among those susceptible at the start of the epidemic. Dashed curves: confidence bounds $\widehat{R} - 2\,\mathrm{s.e.}(\widehat{R})$ and $\widehat{R} + 2\,\mathrm{s.e.}(\widehat{R})$ when ns_0, the number of susceptibles at the start of the epidemic, is 100.*

The solid curve in Figure 8.5 shows the estimate $\widehat{R}$ obtained from (8.2) for different values of y_{S}. The parameter R has been furnished with a "hat" to remind us that we are using Equation (8.2) as a way to provide an estimate of R from the value of y_{S} observed in a specific epidemic.

In Section 8.10.5 we show that a model which allows for randomness also leads to this estimate when the initial number of susceptible community members is large. An advantage of the stochastic model is that it also provides a measure of the precision of the estimate. The large-sample standard error of the estimate $\widehat{R}$ is found to be

$$\mathrm{s.e.}(\widehat{R}) = \frac{1}{\sqrt{ns_0 y_{\mathrm{S}}(1 - y_{\mathrm{S}})}}.$$

The dashed curves in Figure 8.5 show the lower and upper bounds of approximate 95% confidence intervals for any observed attack rate y_S, when $ns_0 = 100$. It is seen that the width of the confidence interval is relatively constant over a large range of observed attack rates, becoming wider when the observed attack rate y_S is small or approaches 1. The width of the confidence interval decreases as ns_0 increases indicating that a precise estimate of R is obtained when the attack rate is from an epidemic with a large number of initial susceptibles.

8.7 Types of individual

It is necessary to allow for types of individual when identifiable groups of people differ in their transmission characteristics. The source of these differences might be behavioral or biological. A difference in immunity status, determined by vaccination status and history of exposure to the infectious disease, is particularly relevant when developing plans for infectious disease control.

8.7.1 Type-specific distribution of cases in an epidemic

To allow for different types of individual we need to allow the transmission intensity between an infective and a susceptible to depend on their type. Consider two types of individual, Type 1 and Type 2, in a large community with $n+1$ members and no household structure. Table 8.1 shows the notation for the type-specific transmission intensity between a given infective and a given susceptible. The functions $\omega_1(u)$ and $\omega_2(u)$ are type-specific infectivity profiles, so the total area under each of their graphs is 1. Differences in the values of β_{11}, β_{12}, β_{21} and β_{22} reflect differences in biological infectivity and susceptibility, as well as differences in the rates of social mixing.

Table 8.1: *Transmission intensity between a given infective and a given susceptible, u days after the infective is infected*

	Type 1 Susceptible	Type 2 Susceptible
Type 1 Infective	$\frac{1}{n}\beta_{11}\omega_1(u)$	$\frac{1}{n}\beta_{12}\omega_1(u)$
Type 2 Infective	$\frac{1}{n}\beta_{21}\omega_2(u)$	$\frac{1}{n}\beta_{22}\omega_2(u)$

By extending the arguments of Section 8.10.1 to two types of individual, we can derive the final-size equations

$$\begin{aligned} 1 - y_{S1} &= \exp[-\beta_{11}s_{01}y_{S1} - \beta_{21}s_{02}y_{S2}] \\ \text{and} \qquad 1 - y_{S2} &= \exp[-\beta_{12}s_{01}y_{S1} - \beta_{22}s_{02}y_{S2}], \end{aligned} \tag{8.3}$$

where y_{S1} is the eventual attack rate among Type 1 susceptibles and s_{01} is the fraction of individuals who are of Type 1 and susceptible at the start of the epidemic, while y_{S2} and s_{02} are the corresponding fractions for Type 2 individuals.

We give two illustrations to show how the final-size equations (8.3) can inform the control of infectious diseases.

8.7.2 Mass vaccination with a partially protective vaccine

Consider a community of homogeneous individuals who are susceptible when a mass vaccination campaign is undertaken. The campaign achieves a coverage of v. When the vaccine offers partial protection, we need to allow for two types of individual, namely unvaccinated individuals (Type 1) and vaccinees (Type 2). In this setting, our definition of type implies that $s_{01} = \tilde{v} = 1 - v$ and $s_{02} = v$.

Attack rates among unvaccinated and vaccinated individual

With a vaccine effect as described in Section 6.1, the two final-size equations become

$$\begin{aligned} 1 - y_{S1} &= \exp(-\beta\,\tilde{v}y_{S1} - b\beta v y_{S2}) \\ \text{and} \qquad & \\ 1 - y_{S2} &= \exp(-a\beta\,\tilde{v}y_{S1} - ab\beta v y_{S2}). \end{aligned} \tag{8.4}$$

For given values of $\beta = R_0$, a and b, we can sketch the graphs of y_{S1}, y_{S2}, $y_1 = \tilde{v}y_{S1}$ and $y_2 = vy_{S2}$ against v. First specify values 0.001, 0.002, ... , 1 for y_{S1} in a spreadsheet. Then calculate the corresponding values of

$$y_{S2} = 1 - (1 - y_{S1})^a \quad \text{and} \quad v = \frac{\ln(1 - y_{S1}) + \beta y_{S1}}{\beta y_{S1} - b\beta y_{S2}}.$$

Figure 8.6 shows the graphs these equations produce with $R_0 = 4$. For graphs in pane A of Figure 8.6 we used $a = 0.1$ and $b = 0.9$, which means that vaccinees have a much reduced susceptibility and an infectivity (in the event of a breakthrough infection) that is reduced by a mere 10%. For graphs in pane B of Figure 8.6 the vaccine-effect parameters are $a = 0.9$ and $b = 0.1$, which means that vaccinees are only marginally less susceptible but vaccinees with a breakthrough infection have low infectivity.

The graphs in Figure 8.6 contain a number of interesting observations. First observe that these two different vaccine responses lead to the same critical vaccination coverage, namely $v^{\dagger} = 0.82$. That is, the attack rates become zero when v reaches the value 0.82. This suggests that a vaccine which induces low susceptibility, but retains high infectivity (here $a = 0.1$ and $b = 0.9$), and a vaccine that reduces susceptibility by a modest amount, but induces low infectivity (here $a = 0.9$ and $b = 0.1$), are equally capable of preventing epidemics. In contrast, we observe that these two vaccine responses show quite different attack rates when the coverage is below the critical vaccination coverage. The combined attack rate in pane A, when

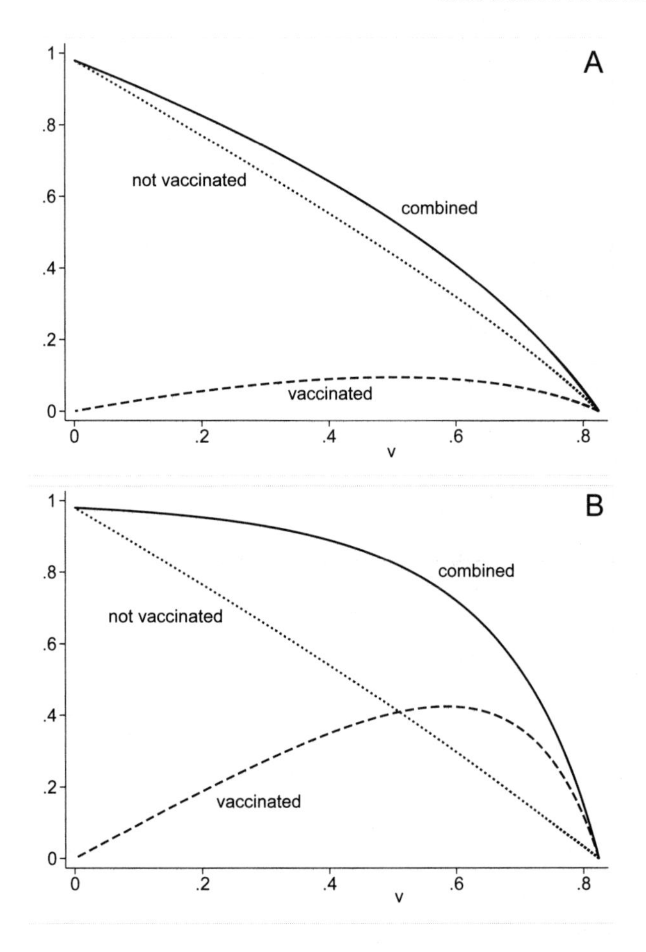

Figure 8.6 *Community attack rates y_1 (unvaccinated), y_2 (vaccinated) and $y = y_1 + y_2$ (combined) for different values of vaccination coverage v, when $R_0 = 4$. In pane A the values of vaccine-effect parameters are $a = 0.1$ and $b = 0.9$ (vaccine is highly protective against infection). In pane B the values of vaccine-effect parameters are $a = 0.9$ and $b = 0.1$ (vaccine reduces infectivity substantially).*

$a = 0.1$ and $b = 0.9$, is lower than the combined attack rate in pane B for all values of v between 0 and 0.82. In particular, when the vaccination coverage is $v = 0.6$ the combined attack rate is $y = 0.72$ in pane B of Figure 8.6, but only 0.41 in pane A of Figure 8.6.

Another interesting observation is the way the fraction of infected individuals who are vaccinees varies as the vaccination coverage is increased. For small values of v nearly all cases are unvaccinated individuals. This is not a surprise because then vaccinees are the smaller group and they are offered some protection by the vaccine. However, as v increases so does the fraction of infected individuals who are vaccinees. This increase may reach the point, as in pane B of Figure 8.6, where the number of infected individuals who are vaccinees exceeds the number who are unvaccinated.

Herd immunity

The way herd immunity was quantified in Section 8.5 can be extended to partially protective vaccines, with the added feature that both unvaccinated individuals and vaccinees benefit from herd immunity. When the vaccine is partially protective, as is often the case, vaccinees acquire some protection against infection from the immune response to their vaccination and acquire further protection, indirectly, from the vaccination of other community members. We illustrate this with an example using the same setting as above, where unvaccinated individuals are Type 1 and vaccinees are Type 2.

Suppose the values of model parameters R_0, a and b are specified, and we are also given the vaccination coverage v. We can then compute the type-specific attack rates y_{S1} and y_{S2}, using Equations (8.4). In the event of an epidemic, $y_{S1} = y_1/(1-v)$ is the probability that an individual, selected randomly from the group of unvaccinated individuals, becomes a case during the epidemic. The indirect immunity acquired by an unvaccinated person is reflected by the reduction in the value of y_{S1} as v is increased. The corresponding probability for an individual selected randomly from vaccinees is $y_{S2} = y_2/v$. The indirect immunity acquired by a vaccinee is reflected by y_{S2} as the vaccination coverage is increased.

Figure 8.7 shows the type-specific attack rates y_{S1}, among unvaccinated individuals, and y_{S2}, among vaccinees, for two different vaccine effects. In both scenarios $R_0 = 4$. For each pair of curves, the amount by which the dashed curve is below the solid curve indicates how much smaller the probability of being infected during the epidemic is for a vaccinee compared to an unvaccinated person, for each specific vaccination coverage v. Note that all curves decline as v is increased. The increasing rate of this decline as v increases, in each curve, shows the indirect protection that mass immunization provides for the corresponding individual. That is, both unvaccinated and vaccinated community members acquire this indirect protection against infection. The rate at which individuals acquire herd immunity is highest as v approaches the critical vaccination coverage, where it is higher for unvaccinated individuals than it is for vaccinees.

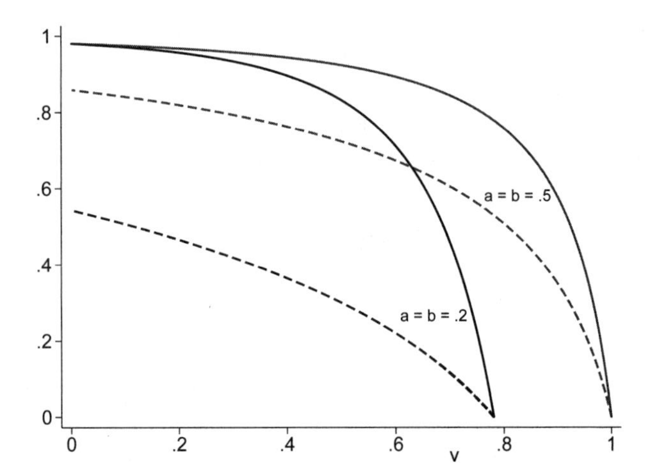

Figure 8.7 *Type-specific attack rates for unvaccinated individuals (y_{S1}, solid curve) and for vaccinees (y_{S2}, dashed curve) for two vaccine effects over different values of the vaccination coverage v, for an infectious disease with $R_0 = 4$. The attack rate gives the probability that an individual of that type is among those infected in the epidemic. The pair of curves with the larger vaccine effect (specified by $a = b = 0.2$) has critical vaccination coverage $v^\dagger = 0.78$, while the pair of curves with the lower vaccine effect (specified by $a = b = 0.5$) has critical vaccination coverage $v^\dagger = 1$.*

8.7.3 Mass immunization to protect a vulnerable group

For a second illustration of the way the final-size equations (8.3) can provide insight we consider a community partitioned into vulnerable individuals (Type 1) and all others (Type 2). For example, the vulnerable group might be the elderly members of the community if the illness they acquire from the infection tends to be much more severe than it is for younger community members. Suppose all community members are susceptible to the infectious disease when a vaccination campaign, achieving a coverage of v, is conducted.

The question is: What distribution of vaccinations over the two types achieves the smallest number of cases in the vulnerable group in a subsequent epidemic? The question arises because, on the one hand, it seems good to vaccinate vulnerable individuals because it protects these immunized individuals fully from severe illness. On the other hand, it may be that Type 2 individuals are the main players in the transmission of the infection. Then it might be better to focus on immunizing Type 2 community members in order to reduce the epidemic size substantially and thereby partially protect *all* vulnerable community members through herd immunity. The best approach depends on many factors, and equations like (8.3) provide a very useful tool to help us answer this question.

For our illustration we assume that

(i) one half of the individuals are Type 1 and the other half are Type 2,
(ii) the transmission parameters in Equations (8.3) are given by $\beta_{11} = 1$, $\beta_{12} = \beta_{21} = 2$ and $\beta_{22} = 4$,
(iii) the vaccine is fully protective, and
(iv) at best, we are able to achieve a vaccination coverage of 50%.

We consider whether it is better to vaccinate only Type 1 individuals or only Type 2 individuals when our aim is to have the smallest number of Type 1 cases in the event of an epidemic.

Vaccinating only Type 1 individuals

With the above parameter values and vaccination restricted to Type 1 individuals the type-specific final-size equations (8.3) become

$$1 - y_{S1} = \exp\left[-(0.5 - v)y_{S1} - y_{S2}\right]$$

and

$$1 - y_{S2} = \exp\left[-(1 - 2v)y_{S1} - 2y_{S2}\right].$$

These equations enable us to sketch the graph of $y_1 = (0.5 - v)y_{S1}$, the attack rate of interest, against v. First specify values 0.001, 0.002, ... , 1 for y_{S2} in one column of a spreadsheet. Then calculate the corresponding values of

$$y_{S1} = 1 - (1 - y_{S2})^{1/2},$$

and

$$v = \frac{\ln(1 - y_{S2}) + y_{S1} + 2y_{S2}}{2y_{S1}}.$$

The dashed curve in Figure 8.8 gives the graph of $y_1 = (0.5 - v)y_{S1}$, the fraction of community members that become vulnerable cases in an epidemic, against the achieved vaccination coverage v.

Vaccinating only Type 2 individuals

If we vaccinate only Type 2 individuals the type-specific final-size equations (8.3) become

$$1 - y_{S1} = \exp\left[-0.5y_{S1} - (1 - 2v)y_{S2}\right]$$

and

$$1 - y_{S2} = \exp\left[-y_{S1} - (2 - 4v)y_{S2}\right].$$

These equations enable us to sketch the graphs of the attack rates against v for this mass vaccination scenario. Insert the values 0.001, 0.002, ... , 1 for y_{S1} in one column of a spreadsheet. Then calculate the corresponding values of

$$y_{S2} = 1 - (1 - y_{S1})^2$$

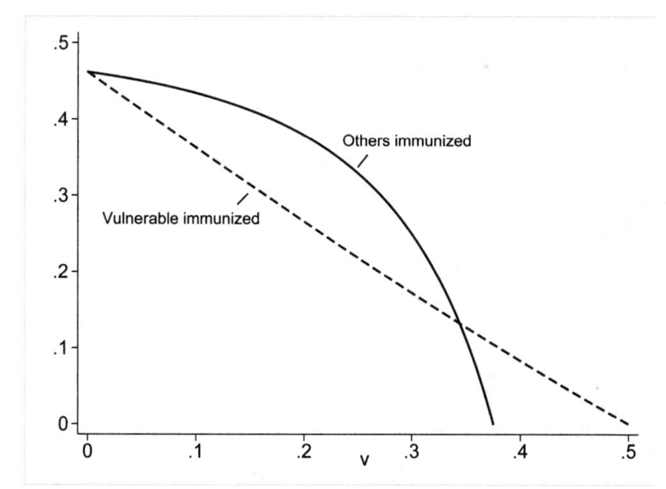

Figure 8.8 *Graphs of y_1, the fraction individuals who are vulnerable and become infected in an epidemic.*

and

$$v = \frac{\ln(1 - y_{S2}) + y_{S1} + 2y_{S2}}{4y_{S2}}.$$

The solid curve in Figure 8.8 gives the graph of $y_1 = 0.5y_{S1}$, the fraction of community members that become vulnerable cases in an epidemic, against the achieved vaccination coverage v.

A comparison of the two curves in Figure 8.8 shows the interesting fact that when the aim is to minimize the number of infections in the vulnerable group it is best to vaccinate members of the vulnerable group if the achievable vaccination coverage is below 34% and it is better to vaccinate non-vulnerable members when the achievable vaccination coverage is above 34%. This dichotomy occurs because the non-vulnerable group plays a larger role in the spread and it is possible to curb this spread sufficiently if the vaccination coverage is high enough.

8.7.4 Parameter estimation

In Section 8.6 we proposed the use of the deterministic final-size equation (8.1) as an estimating equation for the initial reproduction number. This suggests that the type-specific final-size equations (8.3) can be used similarly. This is true *in part* only. It is not entirely true because when we substitute observed attack rates for an epidemic into Equations (8.3) we have two equations with four unknown parameters, namely β_{11}, β_{12}, β_{21} and β_{22}. A solution is only possible when we reduce the number of unknown parameters to two by specifying two independent relationships between these parameters. This is a common problem for multitype models for the spread of infectious diseases.

8.8 Discussion

As always, we must remain aware of the assumptions that lead to our results. For example, the final size equations (8.1) and (8.3) assume that the final size of an epidemic is not appreciably affected by plausible differences in between-household and within-household transmission intensities, nor by any changes in mixing behaviour or public health interventions during the course of the epidemic.

Our modeling approach

It is useful to give an overview of the basic components of our model for the size of an outbreak. Figure 8.9 depicts our two-arm model for the size of the outbreak when the infection is newly introduced into the community.

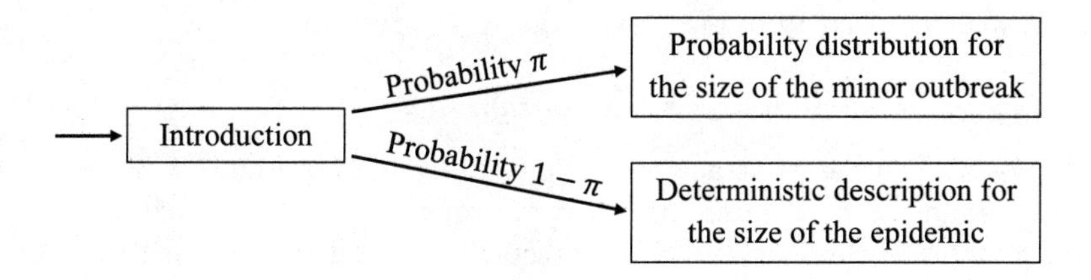

Figure 8.9 *Overview of the model for outbreak size of an introduced infection.*

We began by observing that when an infectious disease is introduced into a community the outcome is certain to be a minor outbreak when R, the initial reproduction number, is less than 1. That is, $R < 1$ implies $\pi = 1$. Then only the upper arm in Figure 8.9 is needed and a stochastic model is used to describe epidemic size. A stochastic model is needed because chance plays a substantial role while the number of infectives is small.

When $R > 1$ there is a chance that the outcome will be a minor outbreak and a chance that an epidemic will occur. Then we need the two arms of the model, allowing chance to determine which model arm is appropriate for any new introduction of the infection. To describe this dichotomy we need the two arms of the model, allowing chance to determine which model arm is appropriate for any new introduction of the infection.

In the lower arm a deterministic model is used to describe the fraction of community members that are infected when an epidemic occurs. The element of chance is less crucial when describing epidemic size because the number of infectives is mostly large during an epidemic. The deterministic model gives an equation that can be solved to give the central value for the epidemic size. This provides a relatively convenient way to gain insights about infectious disease control.

Herd immunity

Figure 8.10 on page 147 shows that the rate of change in y with respect to vaccination coverage v is always less than -1 and becomes -2 as the threshold coverage is approached. This means that every vaccine administered prevents, on average, more than one case in the event of an epidemic and is able to prevent close to two cases when the vaccination coverage is near its threshold value. However, preventing close to two cases per vaccine can be achieved only when susceptibles can be targeted for vaccination. In practice it may not be clear who is susceptible and some immune individuals may be amongst those vaccinated.

We discussed herd immunity in terms of indirect immunity acquired when other community members are vaccinated, because that is relevant to the planning of infectious disease control. Of course, similar indirect immunity is acquired by individuals when other community members have immunity that was acquired from prior exposure to the infection.

Reduced susceptibility versus reduced infectivity

The dotted curves of attack rate in panes A and B of Figure 8.6 show that the amount of herd immunity an unvaccinated individual acquires when the vaccine lowers susceptibility substantially and lowers infectivity by a modest amount is similar to the amount of herd immunity he acquires when vaccine lowers infectivity substantially and lowers susceptibility by a modest amount.

In contrast, the dashed curves in panes A and B of Figure 8.6 tell a different story. When the vaccination uptake is inadequate to prevent an epidemic, a vaccinee can acquire substantially more protection from a vaccine that lowers susceptibility substantially. A lower susceptibility also has a lower combined attack rate (solid curves). This supports a focus on reducing susceptibility when developing a vaccine. This focus is further supported by the fact that a vaccine offering a lower susceptibility is likely to achieve a higher level of uptake than a vaccine offering primarily low infectivity.

8.9 Exercises

1. Suppose the basic reproduction number of an infectious disease in a large community of homogeneous individuals, who mix uniformly, is $R_0 = 4.6$. The community is currently free of the infection. From a large number of blood specimens, it is estimated that 55% of individuals have acquired immunity from previous exposures to the infection. Assume that the offspring distribution for each infective is Poisson.

(a) Suppose one randomly selected individual from the community briefly visits friends outside the community, where he has numerous close contacts with infectives.

Estimate the probability that the individual is infected on his visit.

(b) Suppose one individual is infected when he briefly visits friends outside the community. He returns to spend all of his infectious period circulating, as normal, in his home community.

(i) What is the mean number of individuals this primary infective infects?

(ii) Estimate the probability that this primary infective infects no one.

(iii) Find the probability that this primary infective initiates an epidemic.

(iv) What fraction of the community would be infected if this introduction leads to an epidemic?

(v) Compute the probability that a given susceptible is infected in any transmission subsequent to the introduction of the infection by the primary infective.

2. A new vaccine has been developed to control a certain infectious disease. The vaccine is expensive, but is known to render vaccinees fully protected against infection. Suppose you are a health officer given the task of assessing the likely cost and benefit to the community of an immunization campaign using this vaccine.

Preliminary investigation and analysis of data from your community, from the vaccine manufacturer and from epidemics that occurred in similar communities, yields the following information:

- the basic reproduction number is $R_0 = 6.4$,
- the fraction of your community that is susceptible is $s_0 = 0.4$,
- the cost is \$625,000 for each 1% of your community vaccinated,
- the cost of an epidemic is \$825,000 for each 1% of your community infected.

To continue your investigation make the following calculations.

(a) Compute the fraction of the community that becomes infected if no immunization campaign is conducted and an introduction of the infectious disease leads to an epidemic.

(b) Determine the critical vaccination coverage, i.e., the vaccination coverage required to bring the effective reproduction number down to 1, if the vaccine is administered

(i) to community members independently of their immunity status,

(ii) only to susceptible community members.

(c) To compare costs of different strategies, compute the cost incurred

(i) when no one is vaccinated and an epidemic occurs,

(ii) by an immunization campaign designed to prevent an epidemic by vaccinating community members independently of their immunity status, and

(iii) by an immunization campaign designed to prevent an epidemic by vaccinating only susceptible community members, assuming that the additional total cost of determining the immunity status of every community member is $6,750,000.

(d) Discuss the relative merits of not having an immunization campaign, conducting a campaign that administers the vaccine indiscriminately or conducting a campaign that determines who is susceptible and administers the vaccine only to susceptibles.

3. Two separate uniformly mixing communities, A and B, are currently free from a certain infectious disease. The basic reproduction number for this infection differs in the two communities, because their mixing rates differ. Some individuals acquired immunity from earlier exposure.

   The following is known about the two communities:

	Community A	Community B
Population size	1,200,000	2,500,000
Basic reproduction number	5.2	4.8
Fraction immune	0.74	0.82

(a) For Community A:

(i) Predict the number of cases that would occur if a new introduction leads to an epidemic.

(ii) Determine the number of vaccinations, with a fully protective vaccine, required to prevent an epidemic if

1. vaccines are administered indiscriminately, without reference to immunity status,
2. immunity status is determined and vaccines are administered only to susceptibles.

(b) For Community B:

(i) Compute the mean number of cases in an outbreak initiated by a single, newly infected community member.

(ii) Determine the critical immunity coverage.

4. To protect members of a large uniformly mixing community against a certain infectious disease, 85% of individuals are vaccinated and all unvaccinated individuals are fully susceptible. Vaccination with an active vaccine renders the vaccinee fully protected. In storage, the vaccine may become inactive when it is not maintained in the required temperature range over the period from manufacture until it is used for vaccination. Assume an individual remains fully susceptible when vaccinated with an inactive.

A fresh introduction of this infectious disease leads to an epidemic in which the community attack rate is 0.12 and 20% of the cases are vaccinees. Estimate

(a) f, the proportion of vaccinations that failed to impart immunity,
(b) R_0, the basic reproduction number of the infection in this community,
(c) the effective reproduction number at the start of the outbreak, and
(d) the effective reproduction number at the end of the outbreak.

5. In a uniformly mixing community all individuals are fully susceptible to a certain infection when a vaccination campaign is conducted, achieving a vaccination coverage of $v = 0.76$ with a vaccine offering partial protection. The basic reproduction number is known to be $R_0 = 3.7$. Vaccination reduces the per-contact susceptibility of a vaccinee with a breakthrough infection by a factor a. Vaccination also reduces the transmission intensity exerted by a vaccinee, when he acquires a breakthrough infection, by a factor b when compared to an unvaccinated infective.

   Suppose a post-campaign introduction of the infectious disease leads to an epidemic with a community attack rate of 0.22. Of the epidemic cases 45% are vaccinees. Estimate

   (a) the vaccine effectiveness parameters a and b, and

   (b) the critical immunity coverage for this vaccine.

6. In preparedness planning for the emergence of pandemic influenza, consideration is given to banning mass-gathering events as a way to curb the spread of pandemic influenza. A health officer begins his assessment of this intervention with some simple calculations based on the type-specific attack rate model (8.3), where Type 1 individuals rarely attend mass-gathering events and Type 2 individuals attend them regularly. He reduces the number of parameters by the assumption

$$\begin{pmatrix} \beta_{11} & \beta_{12} \\ \beta_{21} & \beta_{22} \end{pmatrix} = \begin{pmatrix} \alpha & \alpha \\ \alpha & \alpha + \beta \end{pmatrix},$$

   where α and β relate to transmission occurring in general mixing and at mass-gathering events, respectively.

   Suppose it is known that 20% of individuals attend mass-gathering events regularly.

   Compute the type-specific attack rates y_{S1} and y_{S2}, the combined community attack rate y and the type-specific reproduction number R_T when

   (a) $\alpha = 1$ and $\beta = 4$ (no ban on mass-gathering events), and
   (b) $\alpha = 1$ and $\beta = 0$ (total ban on mass-gathering events).

   Comment on the comparison of the results for (a) and (b).

8.10 Supplementary material

8.10.1 Deterministic formula for epidemic size

Consider a large community of homogeneous individuals who mix uniformly. Our aim is to determine the relationship between y, R_0 and s_0, where

R_0 = basic reproduction number,
s_0 = fraction of individuals who are susceptible when the epidemic starts,
y = fraction of community members eventually infected when an epidemic is initiated by a contact with an external infective.

We measure time from the introduction of the infectious disease. The number of individuals infected by time t is denoted $N(t)$ and $S(t) = S(0) - N(t)$ is the number of susceptibles remaining at time t.

Intuitive derivation

We begin with an intuitive look at the relationship between y, R_0 and s_0. Suppose a susceptible individual A is exposed to an aggregated transmission intensity $\lambda(t)$ at time t. That is, $\lambda(t)$ is the transmission intensity obtained when we sum the transmission intensities exerted on A by each individual who is infectious at time t. Now accumulate this aggregated transmission intensity over time points from the start until the end of the epidemic, assumed to occur at time τ. This accumulated aggregated transmission intensity is $\Lambda = \int_0^\tau \lambda(t)\, dt$, the area under the function $\lambda(t)$ over the epidemic period.

By analogy with Equation (5.4), see also Section 5.6.2, the probability that A avoids infection when exposed to this accumulated transmission intensity is $\exp(-\Lambda)$. Therefore $S(\tau)$, the number of community members expected to be susceptible at the end of the epidemic, is

$$S(\tau) \;=\; S(0)\exp(-\Lambda).$$

When the transmission intensity exerted on A by a single infective is accumulated over the entire epidemic period we obtain $\frac{1}{n}R_0$. Summing over all individuals infected during the course of the epidemic leads to $\Lambda = R_0 y$ and

$$s_0 - y \;=\; s_0 \exp(-R_0 y), \tag{8.5}$$

where $y = [S(0) - S(\tau)]/n$ is the eventual attack rate and $s_0 = S(0)/n$ is the fraction of community members initially susceptible.

This intuitive derivation of Equation (8.5) is not convincing in a stochastic setting, because susceptibles do not avoid infection independently. However, this formula does hold in a deterministic formulation, where independence and correlation have no role.

An alternative way to write (8.5) is

$$1 - y_{\mathrm{s}} \;=\; \exp(-R y_{\mathrm{s}}), \tag{8.6}$$

where $y_{\rm S} = y/s_0$ is the eventual attack rate among individuals who are susceptible at the start of the epidemic and $R = R_0 s_0$ is the effective reproduction number at the start of the epidemic.

A more formal derivation

Let the community consist of n susceptibles and one newly infected individual at time $t = 0$. The aggregated transmission intensity acting on each susceptible individual at time t is $\frac{1}{n}\int_0^t \psi(t-x)dN(x)$. Summing this over the number of susceptibles remaining gives the transmission intensity acting on susceptibles, collectively, at time t to be $\int_0^t \psi(t-x)dN(x)\frac{S(t)}{n}$.

In a stochastic model formulation this means that for events in the small time increment $(t, t+dt)$

$$\begin{aligned}\Pr[N(t+dt) = N(t)+1] &\approx \int_0^t \psi(t-x)dN(x)\frac{S(t)}{n}\,.\,dt,\\ \Pr[N(t+dt) = N(t)] &\approx 1 - \int_0^t \psi(t-x)dN(x)\frac{S(t)}{n}\,.\,dt,\end{aligned}$$

and the probability of more than one infection in $(t, t+dt)$ is negligible. These are conditional probabilities, given the transmission process prior to time t.

From these probabilities we deduce that the mean number of infections in $(t, t+dt)$ is $\int_0^t \psi(t-x)dN(x)\frac{S(t)}{n}\,dt$. In a deterministic model formulation this mean is taken as the actual incremental amount by which $N(t)$ is increased, and $S(t)$ is decreased, over the time interval $(t, t+dt)$. That is, the incremental amount by which the number of susceptibles is changed is

$$dS(t) = -\int_0^t \psi(t-x)dN(x)\frac{S(t)}{n}\,.\,dt.$$

Dividing both sides by $S(t)$ and integrating over time gives

$$\int_0^\tau \frac{dS(t)}{S(t)} = \ell n[S(\tau)] - \ell n[S(0)] = -\frac{1}{n}\int_0^\tau \int_0^t \psi(t-x)dN(x)\,dt.$$

When τ is the time when all infection comes to an end, the double integral on the right-hand side of this equation is the aggregation of the transmission intensity function over every individual who became infected and over time from the start of the epidemic until the end of the epidemic. Therefore the right-hand side may be written

$$-\frac{1}{n}R_0\,[S(0) - S(\tau)].$$

Substituting this gives

$$S(\tau) = S(0)\exp\left[-R_0\,\frac{S(0)-S(\tau)}{n}\right]$$

for the eventual number of susceptibles remaining. Dividing both sides by n gives the final-size equation (8.5).

8.10.2 Deterministic version of the transmission threshold property

The curves defined by the left- and right-hand sides of the deterministic final-size equation (8.6), namely

$$1 - y_S = \exp(-Ry_S),$$

intersect at a positive value for y_S only if $R = R_0 s_0 > 1$. Therefore, according to this equation a positive fraction of community individuals is infected if, and only if, $R > 1$.

When $R \leq 1$ the only non-negative solution to the deterministic final-size equation is $y_S = 0$.

8.10.3 Change in the attack rate as the vaccination coverage increases

Suppose that an immunization campaign is implemented in a fully susceptible community, with a vaccine that provides full protection against infection. Then $s_0 = 1 - v$, where v is the vaccination coverage achieved. We are interested in how attack rates y and y_S change as v increases.

A graph of y against the vaccination coverage v shows how mass immunization changes the community attack rate. A convenient way to sketch this graph is to solve the epidemic size equation for v, giving

$$v = 1 + \frac{ln(1 - y_S)}{R_0 y_S}. \qquad (8.7)$$

Then fix a value for R_0 and enter values 0, 0.001, 0.002, ... , 1, for y_S, into a spreadsheet. Finally, use Equation (8.7) to compute the corresponding value for v and plot the graph of $y = (1 - v)y_S$ against v in the range $0 < v < 1$. The solid curves in Figure 8.3 were obtained in this way.

Common features of the relationship between y and v for different values of R_0 can be seen from such graphs, but an algebraic analysis can give clearer insights. To this end we find the rate of change of attack rate y with immunization coverage v. Differentiating (8.5), and a little algebra, gives

$$\frac{dy}{dv} = \frac{-y_S^2}{(1 - y_S)ln(1 - y_S) + y_S}.$$

Figure 8.10 gives a graph of this relationship, which shows that the rate of change of attack rate y is always less than -1 and reaches -2 when the attack rate among susceptibles is close to zero, which occurs when the effective reproduction number approaches 1; in other words, when the vaccination coverage approaches its critical value.

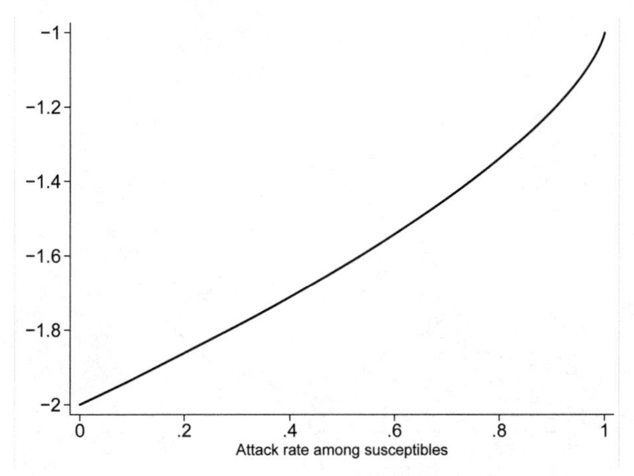

Figure 8.10 *The rate of change in the community attack rate y (with respect to vaccination coverage v) as a function of y_S, the fraction of individuals infected among those susceptible at the start of the epidemic.*

8.10.4 Change in the probability that a susceptible avoids infection

Equation (8.7) can also be used to determine how $1 - y_S$, the probability that a susceptible avoids infection during an epidemic, changes as the immunization coverage is increased.

Differentiating both side of (8.7) with respect to y_S gives

$$\frac{dv}{dy_S} = \frac{-y_S - (1 - y_S)ln(1 - y_S)}{R_0(1 - y_S)y_S^2},$$

and the reciprocal of $\frac{dv}{dy_S}$ is $\frac{dy_S}{dv}$. The three graphs in Figure 8.11 show $\frac{d(1-y_S)}{dv} = -\frac{dy_S}{dv}$ for different values of v when $R_0 = 1.5$, 2.5 and 4. We see that the magnitude of $\frac{d(1-y_S)}{dv}$ increases with v, reaching its maximum as v approaches the critical immunization coverage. To find the rate of change at this point we express the term $ln(1 - y_S)$ in the expression for $\frac{d(1-y_S)}{dv}$ as a Taylor expansion around zero and let $y_S \to 0$. This shows that $\frac{d(1-y_S)}{dv} \to 2R_0$ as $y_S \to 0$.

8.10.5 Estimating R, the initial reproduction number

A convenient way to derive an estimating equation for R from a stochastic model is to use results from martingale theory. Here we outline the argument, omitting technical details.

As mentioned in Section 8.10.1, in a stochastic model we formulate the element of chance with reference to events in small time increments. Let $\mathcal{H}_t$ denote the history of the infection process from 0 to t. Then $dN(t)$,

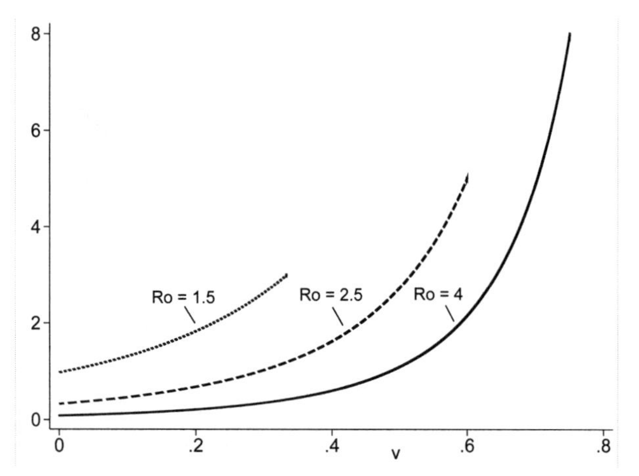

Figure 8.11 *The rate of change of* $1 - y_S$, *the fraction of susceptibles who avoid infection during an epidemic, with respect to* v, *the fraction of immunized community members, for different values of* v.

the change in the number of infections up to time t over the small time increment $(t, t+dt)$, is modeled as

$$\begin{aligned} \Pr[dN(t) = 1 \,|\, \mathcal{H}_t] &= \int_0^t \psi(t-x)dN(x)\frac{S(t)}{n}\,.\,dt, \\ \Pr[dN(t) = 0 \,|\, \mathcal{H}_t] &= 1 - \int_0^t \psi(t-x)dN(x)\frac{S(t)}{n}\,.\,dt, \end{aligned} \tag{8.8}$$

and the probability of more than one infection in $(t, t+dt)$ is taken as negligible. This model formulation implies that

$$\mathrm{E}\left[\frac{1}{S(t)}dN(t)\,\middle|\,\mathcal{H}_t\right] = \frac{1}{n}\int_0^t \psi(t-x)dN(x)\,.\,dt\,.$$

In other words, given the history of the infection process up to time t, the difference

$$\frac{1}{S(t)}dN(t) - \frac{1}{n}\int_0^t \psi(t-x)dN(x)\,.\,dt \tag{8.9}$$

has a mean of zero.

Let τ denote the time when there are no more infectives in the community; that is, the end of the epidemic. If the time interval $(0, \tau)$ is partitioned into a large number of small increments, there is a zero-mean difference like (8.9) for each of them. Summing the zero-mean difference over all the distinct time increments of $(0, \tau)$ gives the expression

$$\int_0^\tau \frac{1}{S(t)}dN(t) - \frac{1}{n}\int_0^\tau \int_0^t \psi(t-x)dN(x)\,dt, \tag{8.10}$$

which has a mean of zero.

The first term in (8.10) is seen to simplify to

$$\int_0^{\tau} \frac{1}{S(0)-N(t))} dN(t) = \frac{1}{S(0)} + \frac{1}{S(0)-1} + \cdots + \frac{1}{S(0)-N(\tau)+1}.$$

For a large community, the sum on the right-hand side is approximately

$$\int_{S(0)-N(\tau)}^{S(0)} \frac{1}{x}\, dx = \ln\left[\frac{S(0)}{S(0)-N(\tau)}\right] = -\ln(1-y/s_0),$$

where $y = N(\tau)/n$ is the community attack rate, and $s_0 = S(0)/n$ is the fraction of the community that is susceptible at the start of the epidemic.

The double integral of (8.10) is the area under the transmission intensity function $\psi(x)$ for each of the $N(\tau)$ individuals infected during the epidemic. That is,

$$\frac{1}{n}\int_0^{\tau}\int_0^{t} \psi(t-x)dN(x)\, dt = \frac{1}{n} N(\tau)R_0 = yR_0.$$

Therefore, by equating the expression (8.10) to zero, its mean, we obtain the estimating equation

$$-\ln(1-y/s_0) - yR_0 = 0.$$

A little algebra allows us to write this as

$$R_0 = \frac{-\ln(1-y/s_0)}{y} \qquad \text{or} \qquad R = \frac{-\ln(1-y_{\mathrm{S}})}{y_{\mathrm{S}}},$$

where $R = R_0 s_0$ is the effective reproduction number at the start of the epidemic and $y_{\mathrm{S}} = N(\tau)/S(0)$.

We see that this stochastic modeling approach leads to the same estimating equation for R as is obtained from the deterministic final-size formula (8.2). The advantage of stochastic modeling is that we can proceed similarly to obtain a standard error for our estimate and then use the Martingale Central Limit Theorem to construct a confidence interval for R.

Given $\mathcal{H}_t$, the history of the infection process up to time t, the only random element in the term (8.9) is $dN(t)$. Therefore, conditional on $\mathcal{H}_t$, its variance is

$$\mathrm{Var}\left[\frac{1}{S(t)} dN(t) - \frac{1}{n}\int_0^t \psi(t-x)dN(x)\,.\,dt \,\Big|\, \mathcal{H}_t\right] = \frac{1}{S^2(t)} \mathrm{Var}[dN(t) \,|\, \mathcal{H}_t].$$

Using probability distribution (8.8) and the fact that $\Pr[dN(t) = 1 \,|\, \mathcal{H}_t]$ is very small gives $\mathrm{Var}[dN(t) \,|\, \mathcal{H}_t] = \mathrm{E}[dN(t) \,|\, \mathcal{H}_t]$. Therefore $dN(t)$ "estimates" $\mathrm{Var}[dN(t) \,|\, \mathcal{H}_t]$ and summing over all the time increments that make up $(0,\tau)$ we find the estimated variation of (8.10) as

$$\begin{aligned}
\int_0^\tau \frac{dN(t)}{[S(t)]^2} &= \frac{1}{[S(0)]^2} + \frac{1}{[S(0)-1]^2} + \cdots + \frac{1}{[S(0)-N(\tau)+1]^2} \\
&\approx \int_{S(0)-N(\tau)}^{S(0)} \frac{1}{x^2}\,dx = \left[-\frac{1}{x}\right]_{S(0)-N(\tau)}^{S(0)} \\
&= \frac{1}{S(0)-N(\tau)} - \frac{1}{S(0)} \\
&= \frac{y}{ns_0(s_0-y)}.
\end{aligned}$$

From Martingale Theory, which we do not elaborate on here, we know that the square root of this variation is the appropriate normalizing factor in the central limit theorem for the zero mean martingale (8.10). Therefore

$$\frac{-\ln(1-y/s_0) - yR_0}{\sqrt{\frac{y}{ns_0(s_0-y)}}} = \sqrt{ns_0y_{\mathrm{S}}(1-y_{\mathrm{S}})}\left[\frac{-\ln(1-y_{\mathrm{S}})}{y_{\mathrm{S}}} - R\right]$$

is approximately a standard Normal variable when an epidemic occurs in a community with a large number of susceptibles at the start of the outbreak. Here $R = R_0s_0$, the effective reproduction number at the start of the outbreak.

In terms of estimation this means that

$$\widehat{R} = \frac{-\ln(1-y_{\mathrm{S}})}{y_{\mathrm{S}}}$$

estimates $R = R_0s_0$ with large-sample standard error

$$\text{s.e.}\big(\widehat{R}\big) = 1\Big/\sqrt{ns_0y_{\mathrm{S}}(1-y_{\mathrm{S}})},$$

and

$$\left[\widehat{R} - 2\,\text{s.e.}\big(\widehat{R}\big),\ \widehat{R} + 2\,\text{s.e.}\big(\widehat{R}\big)\right]$$

is an approximate 95% confidence interval for R.

8.11 Bibliographic notes

The idea of using a two-armed model, like that depicted in Figure 8.9, comes from Kendall (1956). The final-size equation (8.1) is first given in Kermack and McKendrick (1927), while Ma and Earn (2006) examine the generality and limitations of this equation. The large-population final-size distribution for the stochastic epidemic model is derived by von Bahr and Martin-Löf (1980). Britton (1998) discusses parameter estimation for a multitype epidemic model. The martingale methods for infectious disease models used in Section 8.10.5 are reviewed by Becker (1993).

CHAPTER 9

Dynamics of infection incidence

Our discussion of epidemics has so far focussed on the impact of control measures on the probability that an epidemic occurs when an infection is introduced and on the eventual attack rate in the event of an epidemic. When preparing for an epidemic, one is also interested in the effect of control measures on other characteristics of an epidemic. These include

(i) the initial rate of increase in case incidence,
(ii) the case load at the peak of the epidemic, and
(iii) the duration of the epidemic.

To discuss aspects such as these we need ways to study the effect of control measures on the incidence of cases over time.

Models that describe the time dynamics of the transmission of infectious diseases are also needed for the important task of estimating parameters from daily disease incidence data.

9.1 The epidemic curve

Consider a large community that has been free from a certain infection and this infection is then introduced by a contact with an external infective. When the initial R exceeds 1, such an introduction can result in a minor outbreak or an epidemic. Here we assume that an epidemic occurs.

A plot of daily case counts is called an epidemic curve. It provides a convenient visual picture of the progress of the epidemic over time. We describe the temporal progress of epidemic disease transmission by a deterministic model. That is, we construct a model for the epidemic curve that is based on the trend of transmission. It ignores the random fluctuations around this trend that is usually observed in practice.

We look first at an epidemic curve constructed by describing transmission events in successive time increments. This approximates a continuous-time epidemic curve. We then formulate a model for the progression of transmission in "generation time." The latter is often a preferred tool for assessing control measures, because its relatively simple equations can reduce computing time substantially.

9.1.1 Incremental time steps

Consider a uniformly mixing community of size $n + 1$, where n is large. The community has been free from a certain infectious disease when one community member is infected by an external contact. Taking this point of time as our time origin, we consider, in turn, how much new infection occurs in each of the successive time increments $(0, \delta]$, $(\delta, 2\delta]$, $(2\delta, 3\delta]$, $\ldots$, where δ has a small positive value. For example, δ might be 0.1 of a day.

Let $I(j\delta)$ denote the "number of new infections" arising during the period from time $(j-1)\delta$ to time $j\delta$. The plot of $I(\delta)$, $I(2\delta)$, $I(3\delta)$, $\ldots$ against times δ, 2δ, 3δ, $\ldots$, respectively, gives the epidemic curve for infection incidence. The way $I(\delta)$, $I(2\delta)$, $I(3\delta)$, $\ldots$ are computed is described in Section 9.6.1.

Figure 9.1 shows an epidemic curve computed in this way using $n = 1000$, $R_0 = 1.5$, $\delta = 1$ and infectivity profile

$$\omega(u) = \begin{cases} 0.25, & \text{if } 6 \le u \le 10, \\ 0, & \text{otherwise.} \end{cases}$$

The initial waves of infection shown in the curve stem from a latent period that is longer than the infectious period. These waves are gradually dampened out as generations of cases increasingly overlap in calendar time.

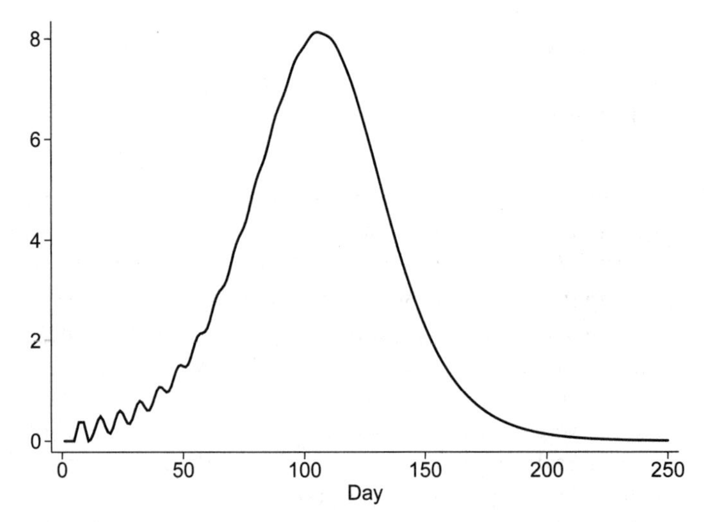

Figure 9.1 *Epidemic curve for an infectious disease in a community with one initial infective and 1000 initial susceptibles when $R_0 = 1.5$ and an individual's infectivity is flat over a period of four days following a latent period of six days.*

This way of computing the epidemic curve is manageable, using a spreadsheet and a little programming. The epidemic curve obtained is close to the continuous-time epidemic model when the value of δ is small. The cost of choosing a small value for δ lies in the amount of computation time, which increases rapidly as δ is decreased. On the other hand, using a value of δ that is too large leads to an approximation that is inadequate for a reliable assessment of the impact of control measures. A time increment of $\delta = 1$ day gives an epidemic curve that is close to the curve for the underlying continuous-time model when R_0 and $\omega(u)$ are as specified for Figure 9.1.

9.1.2 Generation time steps

A simpler approach is to consider the progress of the epidemic in terms of successive generations. Denote the number of infectives in Generation j by I_j, with $I_1 = 1$ corresponding to the initial infective. Let S_1 be the number of community suceptibles exposed to the initial infective.

Each of the S_1 susceptibles, independently, has probability $\exp[-R_0/n]$ of avoiding infection by the initial infective, where R_0 is the basic reproduction number; see Section 5.6.2. In the generation model we determine the number of infectives in Generation 2 by

$$I_2 = S_1[1 - \exp(-R_0 I_1/n)],$$

the mean number of community members infected by the initial infective.

Next, we adjust the number of susceptibles remaining to $S_2 = S_1 - I_2$. Note that I_2 and S_2 are unlikely to be integers. Nevertheless, we think of I_2 and S_2 as "number of individuals" and argue that each of the S_2 susceptibles remaining, independently, has probability $1 - \exp(-R_0 I_2/n)$ of being infected by exposure to the I_2 infectives of Generation 2. The mean number of the S_2 susceptibles infected by a Generation 2 infectives is

$$I_3 = S_2[1 - \exp(-R_0 I_2/n)],$$

which we take as the "number" of cases in Generation 3.

In this way we iteratively compute the "number" of susceptibles remaining and the "number" of cases in each of the generations of the epidemic. The series of $I_1, I_2, I_3, \ldots$ values captures the progress of the epidemic in generations. We can map this series of generation counts to calendar time by locating the I_j cases of Generation j at the calendar time $t_j = (j-1) \times u_{\text{M}}$, where u_{M} is the median of the infectivity profile $\omega(u)$. That is, u_{M} is such that

$$\begin{aligned} \text{area under } \omega(u) \text{ to the left of } u_{\text{M}} &= \text{area under } \omega(u) \text{ to the right of } u_{\text{M}} \\ &= 0.5. \end{aligned}$$

Figure 9.2 is the bar graph of an "epidemic curve" computed in this way using $n = S_1 = 1000$, $R_0 = 1.5$ and $u_{\text{M}} = 8$, which corresponds to the setting used for Figure 9.1.

The transmission progress depicted in Figure 9.1 and Figure 9.2 shows a

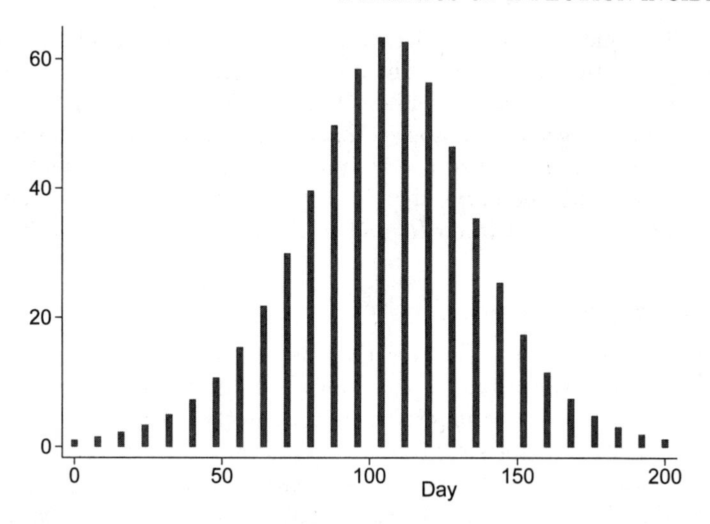

Figure 9.2 *Bar graph of the "epidemic curve" in generation time for an infectious disease in a community with one initial infective and 1000 initial susceptibles, when* $R_0 = 1.5$ *and the median of the infectivity profile is eight days.*

very similar pattern. Note, however, that the vertical axes of the two graphs have a different scale. This difference arises because Figure 9.1 shows the increase in the number of individuals infected so far on a day-by-day basis, whereas Figure 9.2 shows the increase in the number infected over an eight-day period. For a direct comparison of the two curves we divide the I_j of Figure 9.2 by 8 and allocate the resulting number of cases to each of the eight days that make up the eight-day period. This gives the histogram shown in Figure 9.3. Superimposed on this histogram is the epidemic curve of Figure 9.1.

We see that the match of the two epidemic curves is very good, suggesting that the epidemic curve derived from the generations can confidently be used to study the impact of control measures on key characteristics of the epidemic curve. This is extremely useful because calculations based on the generation time model are much easier to set up and less computer intensive.

9.2 Estimating parameter values from daily incidence data

Emergence of a new infectious disease, or reappearance of an infection with a high incidence of severe illness, tends to trigger a period of enhanced surveillance. Timely data on daily incidence counts become available, making it possible to obtain a timely estimate of the initial reproduction number R, and possibly other model parameters. These early estimates, used in models, help to guide management of the epidemic.

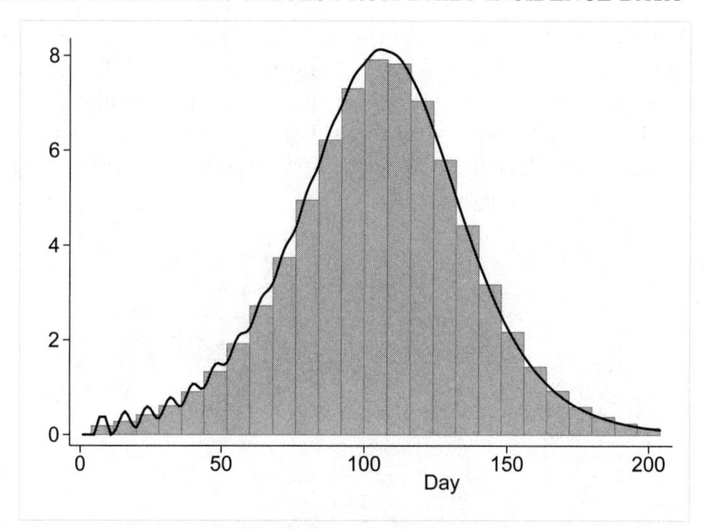

Figure 9.3 *Comparison of the epidemic curves from Figure 9.1 and Figure 9.2 using a common scale on the vertical axis.*

In Section 2.7.1 we used daily case incidence over the initial stage of an epidemic to estimate R, by identifying generations of infectives. That approach requires generations to be unambiguously identifiable during the early stage of the epidemic. We now describe an approach that can estimate R and characteristics of the infectivity profile, simultaneously, using daily incidence when initial generations overlap to some extent. Roughly speaking, we use the initial rise in the epidemic curve and initial fluctuations in this curve, such as those seen in Figure 9.1, to estimate model parameters.

9.2.1 Maximum likelihood estimation using only daily incidence

Consider an outbreak of a newly introduced infectious disease in a large community. Let Day 1 be the day when symptomatic cases are first observed. We describe a method to estimate model parameters under the following assumptions:

(i) each infective has the same infectivity profile,
(ii) infectives infect individuals independently, and
(iii) $I(1)$, the number of cases with symptom onset on Day 1, is known.

During the early stage of the outbreak the depletion of susceptible individuals is negligible and we deduce, from the above assumptions, that the number infected by each infective is a random realization from the Poisson offspring distribution with mean R, the initial reproduction number.

We need a little more notation to explain what else our assumptions imply. Suppose individual B is infected by an infective A. Let p_j denote the probability that B shows symptoms j days after onset of symptoms in A. Then the values p_1, p_2, $p_3, \ldots$ specify the probability distribution of the serial interval. Our assumptions imply that the number of offspring generated by A who show symptoms $1, 2, 3, \ldots$ days later is a Poisson variable with mean Rp_1, Rp_2, $Rp_3, \ldots$, respectively (see Figure 9.4). These Poisson variables are independent.

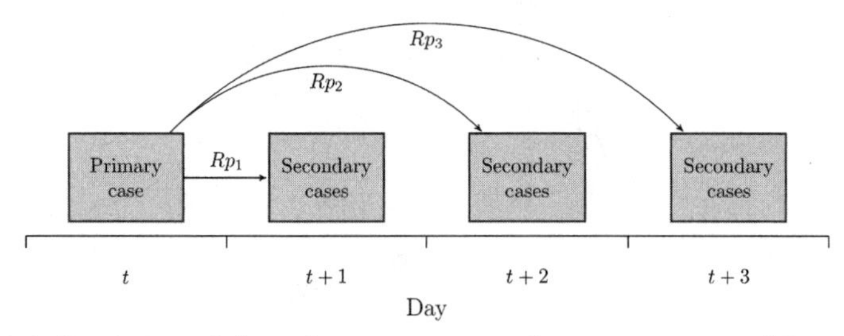

Figure 9.4 *Depiction of day of symptom onset for cases generated by a primary case who became symptomatic on day t.*

Let $I(1)$, $I(2)$, ..., $I(k)$ denote the number of cases with symptom onset on days $1, 2, \ldots, k$, respectively. Under our assumptions the expression for the likelihood function corresponding to observed counts $I(2)$, $I(3)$, ..., $I(k)$ is

$$\ell_1(R, p_1, p_2, \ldots) = \text{constant} \times \mu_2^{I(2)} e^{-\mu_2} \times \mu_3^{I(3)} e^{-\mu_3} \times \cdots \times \mu_k^{I(k)} e^{-\mu_k} \quad (9.1)$$

where

$$\mu_j = [I(1)p_{j-1} + I(2)p_{j-2} + I(3)p_{j-3} \cdots + I(j-1)p_1]R.$$

Daily incidences contain only a limited amount of information about the serial interval, so some constraint on the p_1, p_2, $p_3, \ldots$ is required. As is common in statistical inference, we specify a parametric form for the probability distribution of the serial interval, so that only one or two parameters need to be estimated to specify the p_j. For example, suppose the serial interval has a Weibull distribution specified by probability density function

$$f(u; \alpha, \beta, \gamma) = \begin{cases} 0, & \text{if } 0 \le u < \gamma, \\ \frac{\alpha}{\beta}\left(\frac{u-\gamma}{\beta}\right)^{\alpha-1} \exp\left[-\left(\frac{u-\gamma}{\beta}\right)^{\alpha}\right], & \text{if } u \ge \gamma. \end{cases}$$

For a random variable U with this distribution we find

$$\Pr(U > u) = \begin{cases} 1, & \text{if } 0 \le u < \gamma, \\ \exp\left[-\left(\frac{u-\gamma}{\beta}\right)^{\alpha}\right], & \text{if } u \ge \gamma. \end{cases} \quad (9.2)$$

The p_1, p_2, $p_3, \ldots$ are the day-by-day probabilities of this distribution, given by

$$p_j = \Pr(j-1 < U \leq j) = \Pr(U > j-1) - \Pr(U > j)$$

This expresses every p_j in terms of α, β and γ. We may be able to use existing knowledge to assign a value to one or two of theses parameters and can then estimate the remaining parameter(s) using the likelihood function (9.1).

Application to smallpox data

To illustrate this method for estimating parameters and, specifically, to demonstrate that daily incidence counts for the early days of an epidemic enable estimation of some characteristics of the serial interval we apply the approach to the smallpox data shown in Figure 2.5. The daily incidence counts are shown in Table 9.1 for days with new cases. The days in-between had no new cases.

Table 9.1: *Incidence counts on days with variola minor cases*

Day	1	17	18	19	20	31	33	35	45	48	52	54	55	56
Cases	1	1	1	2	1	1	1	1	1	2	1	4	1	1
Day	57	58	59	66	67	69	70	71	72	73	74	76	78	85
Cases	1	1	1	1	1	2	2	3	4	2	5	2	2	1

For this application we base the distribution for the serial interval on the Weibull distribution (9.2). To keep the illustration simple we set the parameter values $\alpha = 2$ and $\gamma = 12$, leaving parameters R and β to be estimated from the data. Specifically, we have assumed a latent period of 12 days for smallpox. This choice of Weibull distribution gives

$$p_j = \begin{cases} 0, & \text{if } j = 1, 2, \ldots, 12, \\ \exp\left[-\left(\frac{j-13}{\beta}\right)^2\right] - \exp\left[-\left(\frac{j-12}{\beta}\right)^2\right], & \text{if } j = 13, 14, 15, \ldots . \end{cases}$$

To find the maximum likelihood estimates of β and R, we need to find the values of β and R for which the likelihood (9.1) assumes its largest value. For this task we can choose the constant in (9.1) to be any value that is convenient. Once we specify values for β and R we can compute, in turn, all the p_j values and all the μ_j values. Substituting these values into Equation (9.1) gives the value of the likelihood function $\ell_1(R, p_1, p_2, \ldots)$ corresponding to the selected values of β and R. This enables us to find the maximum likelihood estimates of β and R, with the aid of a spreadsheet.

In this way, the data in Table 9.1 give the maximum likelihood estimates $\hat{\beta} = 7.1$ and $\hat{R} = 1.9$. Note that this estimate of R is similar to the estimate obtained in Section 2.7.1.

To show that the daily incidence data contain information about the probability distribution of the serial interval we have plotted, in Figure 9.5, the profile of the likelihood function over values of β when R is set at the value 1.9. The fact that the profile of likelihood values falls away rapidly on both sides of its maximum value demonstrates that the daily incidences are informative about the distribution of the serial interval.

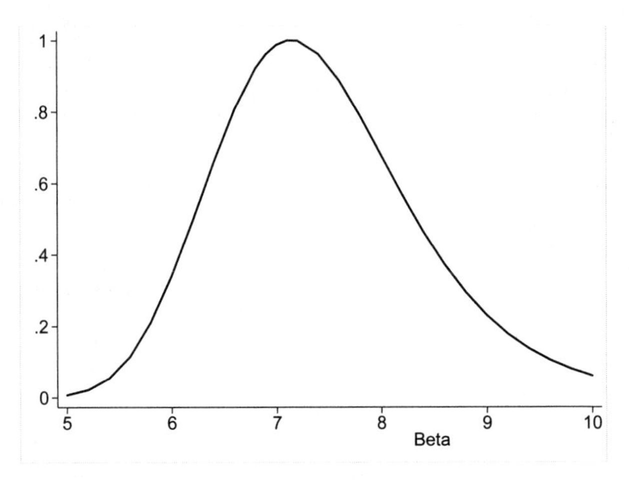

Figure 9.5 *Profile of the likelihood function over values of scale parameter β, given $R = 1.9$. The vertical axis is scaled so that the maximum value of the likelihood is unity.*

The estimate of R is also found to be quite precise. This is seen from Figure 9.6, which shows the profile of the likelihood function over values of R, with $\beta = 7.1$. The rapid drop in values of the likelihood as R moves away from the value 1.9, on both sides, indicates the precision of the estimate of R.

The estimated distribution of the serial interval, obtained by substituting $\hat{\beta} = 7.1$ for β in the expressions for $p_1, p_2, p_3, \ldots$, is shown in Figure 9.7.

In contrast to the method described in Section 2.7.1 for the estimation of R, the present approach does not assume that we can allocate all early cases to generations. It permits some overlap in the early generations, although for precise estimation some clustering of cases should be evident. The method of estimation described here also has the advantage of being able to include data beyond the stage where generations are clearly identifiable. Data for additional days contribute little to the precision of

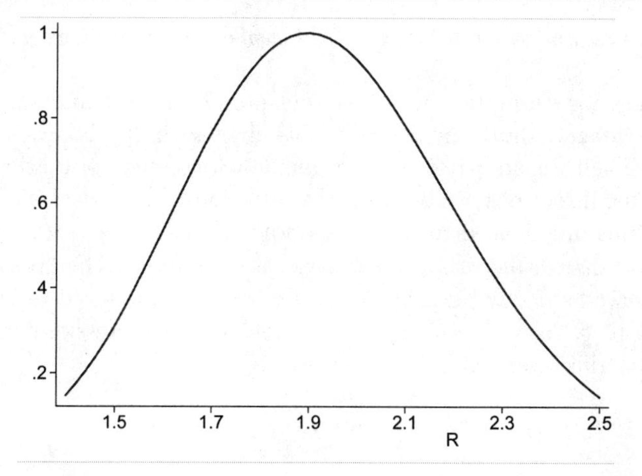

Figure 9.6 *Profile of the likelihood function over values of the initial reproduction number R, given $\beta = 7.1$. The vertical axis is scaled so that the maximum value of the likelihood is unity.*

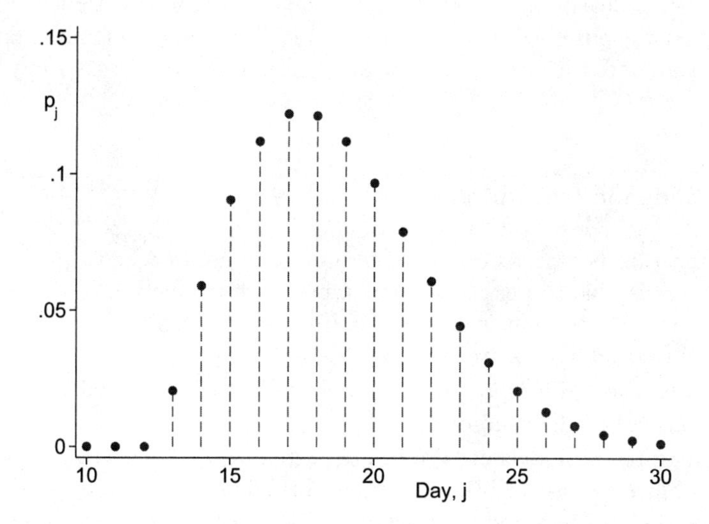

Figure 9.7 *Daily probabilities p_1, p_2, $p_3, \ldots$ for the distribution of the serial interval.*

inferences about the distribution of the serial interval, because generations overlap significantly over the later period. However, data on the additional days can improve the precision of the estimate of R considerably.

9.2.2 Estimation when some serial intervals are observed as well

Sometimes, for example when the latent period is short and the infectious period is longer, daily incidence counts display little, if any, early wave pattern. Then, in addition to daily incidence counts, estimation of R requires some direct observations on the duration of the serial interval. Such observations might arise from contact tracing.

Suppose that, in addition to the incidence counts for the first k days, we have observed some serial intervals. Let r_j of these observed serial intervals be equal to j days, $j = 1, 2, \ldots$. The likelihood corresponding to these observed serial intervals is

$$\ell_2(p_1, p_2, \ldots) = \text{constant} \times p_1^{r_1} \times p_2^{r_2} \times p_3^{r_3} \times \cdots .$$

The full likelihood, corresponding to observed daily case incidences and the observed serial intervals, is then

$$\ell(R, p_1, p_2, \ldots) = \ell_1(R, p_1, p_2, \ldots) \times \ell_2(p_1, p_2, \ldots).$$

We then proceed, as before, by specifying a parametric form for the p_j, inserting the observed data into the full likelihood function and maximizing the likelihood with respect to R and parameters used to specify p_1, p_2, $p_3, \ldots$.

9.3 Endemic transmission

An infection is said to be *endemic* in a community when a positive case incidence is able to persist without repeated introduction of the infection. Endemic transmission is possible only when demographic and infectious disease characteristics are suitable.

Firstly, the basic reproduction number R_0 must exceed 1 for the infectious disease in the community.

According to models used so far, persistent infection necessarily depletes the number of susceptibles, eventually bringing the effective reproduction number below unity and the infection is then certain to be eliminated. This is a consequence of assuming a closed community and a period of immunity for those recovered from infection. Endemic transmission is only possible when new susceptibles are generated. This can occur by births, immigration or waning immunity in individuals previously infected or immunized.

A third requirement for endemic transmission is a large community, because real-world replenishment of susceptibles in a small community, such as a household, a boarding school or a village, is unlikely to match the depletion in susceptibles from endemic transmission of the infection.

9.3.1 Steady incidence of infections

Consider a large community in which an infectious disease has a basic reproduction number $R_0 > 1$ and the pool of susceptibles is steadily refreshed by births, immigrants or waning immunity at a rate that enables endemic transmission to occur. Assume that the incidence of new infections is steady, or fluctuates around a steady rate. This implies that R, the effective reproduction number, is essentially 1. That is, $R = R_0 s_E \simeq 1$, where s_E denotes the fraction of individuals that is susceptible when transmission is endemic. It follows that, when there is steady endemic transmission in a community, the basic reproduction number is given by

$$R_0 = 1/s_E. \tag{9.3}$$

This equation points to possible ways to estimate R_0, which is important for the control of infectious diseases because R_0 determines the fraction of the community that must be immunized, in the long term, to eliminate the infectious disease and prevent future epidemics.

9.3.2 Estimating R_0

One way to estimate R_0 is to insert an estimate of s_E, obtained from serological survey data, into Equation (9.3). The idea is to collect a blood sample from each individual in a random selection of community members and use these to determine the fraction of individuals with antibody levels low enough to leave them susceptible to infection. This is feasible, although such surveys are usually quite costly.

A cheaper and more convenient approach is to use data that are routinely collected. To describe this approach we write (9.3) as

$$R_0 = \frac{\text{number alive}}{\text{number susceptible}}, \tag{9.4}$$

where the numerator and denominator are numbers during steady endemic transmission. Next, we derive expressions for the numerator and denominator in terms of quantities such as age at infection and survival probabilities. Data on these quantities are normally recorded in years. We therefore describe the approach using discrete years as our unit of time.

Suppose susceptibles are replenished by n_0 new births every year and let q_j denote the probability that an individual survives, at least, to the end of the jth year of life. With this notation the numerator in Equation (9.4) can be written in terms of the number in each age year, as

$$\text{number alive} = n_0 q_1 + n_0 q_2 + n_0 q_3 + \cdots . \tag{9.5}$$

The q_j and n_0 are determined accurately from birth and death records. Specifically, the probability q_j can be estimated by the proportion of births observed to survive to the end of the jth year of life.

Using the argument in Section 9.6.2 we write the denominator of (9.4) in terms of the number in each age year and not yet infected, as

$$\text{number susceptible} = n_0 q_1 \mathrm{e}^{-\lambda} + n_0 q_2 \mathrm{e}^{-2\lambda} + n_0 q_3 \mathrm{e}^{-3\lambda} + \cdots , \tag{9.6}$$

where λ is the constant infection intensity exerted on each susceptible individual when transmission is endemic in the community. In Section 9.6.2 we explain that λ is estimated by $1/\bar{a}$, where $\bar{a}$ is the mean of observed ages at the time of infection.

Substituting the expressions (9.5) and (9.6) into Equation (9.4) gives the relationship

$$R_0 = \frac{q_1 + q_2 + q_3 + \cdots}{q_1 \exp(-1/\bar{a}) + q_2 \exp(-2/\bar{a}) + q_3 \exp(-3/\bar{a}) + \cdots} . \tag{9.7}$$

The basic reproduction number can be estimated from this expression by substituting the observed average age at infection $\bar{a}$ and an estimate for each q_j based on the proportion of births observed to survive to the end of the jth year of life.

How R_0 depends on the age at infection

To illustrate the relationship between R_0 and $\bar{a}$ we adopt the form for q_1, q_2, q_3, ... , given by

$$q_j = \begin{cases} 1, & \text{if } j = 1, 2, \ldots, \gamma, \\ \exp\left[-\left(\frac{j-\gamma}{\beta}\right)^{\alpha}\right], & \text{if } j = \gamma+1, \gamma+2, \gamma+3, \ldots . \end{cases} \tag{9.8}$$

This form assumes that mortality is negligible up to the age of γ years. For our illustration we set $\gamma = 60$. The other two parameters are taken as $\alpha = 2.5$ and $\beta = 18$, giving a median age lived of about 75 years and about 4% reaching the age of 90 years. This is broadly consistent with survival in developed nations. Figure 9.8 gives the graph of the survival probabilities $q_{55}, q_{56}, q_{57}, \ldots, q_{100}$ with these parameter values.

When we insert these values for the q_j, expression (9.7) for R_0 depends only on $\bar{a}$. Figure 9.9 shows this relationship. For any observed value of $\bar{a}$ we can use the graph to estimate the value of R_0 for this community. For example, the estimate of R_0 is 6.65 when $\bar{a} = 10$ years is observed.

9.4 Discussion

The models used in this chapter are largely deterministic formulations, which ignore chance fluctuations. As mentioned, deterministic models tend to be more manageable and provide satisfactory descriptions of endemic and epidemic transmission in large communities. However, it is important to be aware of some limitations.

Firstly, although deterministic equations can provide estimates, for ex-

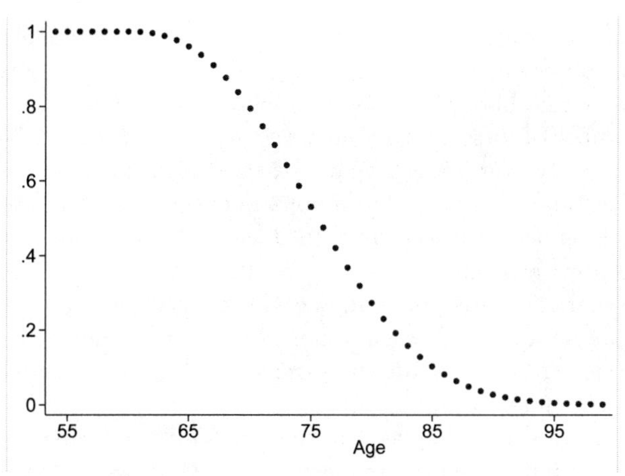

Figure 9.8 *Survival probabilities q_j for ages $j = 55, 56, 57, \ldots$ 100 years, as given by Equation (9.8) with $\alpha = 2.5$, $\beta = 18$ and $\gamma = 60$.*

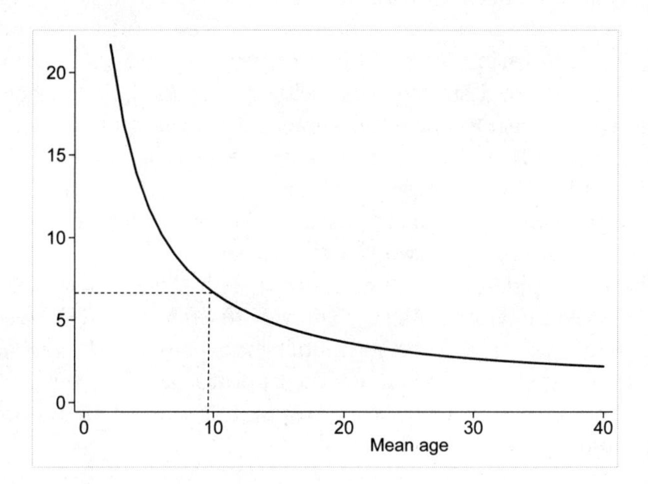

Figure 9.9 *Relationship between R_0 and the mean age at infection, assuming endemic transmission in a population with age distribution shown in Figure 9.8.*

ample by using Equation (9.7), they do not provide an accompanying standard error or other measure of precision for the estimate.

Secondly, the description deterministic models provide of fade-out of the infection from the community requires careful scrutiny. This is not a problem while there is a substantial infection incidence, but can be a problem when the number of infectives reaches low values. We can learn something about fade-out from a deterministic model by looking to see when the number of infectives falls below 1 in the model. However, the number of infectives never actually reaches zero in a deterministic model. The model continues to describe, rather artificially, the dynamics during the time period when the number of infectives is below 1. In reality it is most likely that the number of infectives actually becomes zero during this period and transmission only commences again when the infection is re-introduced from outside the community. As a consequence, a deterministic model is not a reliable indicator of the time until the next outbreak.

Finally, as we have mentioned before, deterministic models do not acknowledge that the outcome of an occasional introduction of the infection may be a minor outbreak even when $R > 1$. We sidestepped this deficiency of a deterministic model by using a deterministic model only when an epidemic actually occurs.

We should point out that assumptions made in this chapter can be relaxed. For example, the method for estimating R_0 described in Section 9.3.2 assumes a fixed number of births each year. This provides a simplification, because n_0 then cancels out and does not appear in expression (9.7) for R_0. However, it is straightforward to derive an expression with the number of births in each of the past years left arbitrary. The resulting expression for R_0 can be used to estimate R_0 if birth records for past years are available.

The assumption of a steady case incidence seems limiting, because real world endemic transmission often shows some seasonality. However, the seasonality is merely a fluctuation around a steady incidence rate and the method for estimating R_0 described in Section 9.3.2 remains sensible provided we estimate the mean age at infection from data collected over a longer time period, such as two years or more.

The observed epidemic curve consists of daily case counts, whereas our model is for new infections. As case counts are essentially a delayed version of counts of infection incidence our model shares most of the characteristics of the case-count curve. When we incorporate an intervention into our model its impact will reflect the corresponding impact in the case-count epidemic curve.

9.5 Exercises

1. Consider epidemics in a uniformly mixing community of homogeneous individuals.
   (a) Explain why, for a closed community, a typical epidemic curve
      (i) rises sharply initially,
      (ii) does not display a flat peak, i.e., a period of near-constant incidence,
      (iii) declines rapidly on the other side of the peak, and
      (iv) shows roughly as many infections during the period when $R < 1$ as occurred during the period when $R > 1$.

(b) Describe a feature of transmission that might explain why some endemic infectious diseases are observed to have epidemic seasons.

(c) Describe a feature of transmission that might explain why an epidemic of a newly emerged infectious disease is not always followed by a period of elimination of the infectious disease.

2. Suppose an epidemic is initiated when one individual is infected with a newly emerged infection just prior to joining a community consisting of 1000 susceptibles. The initial reproduction number is $R_0 = 1.6$ and the infectivity profile is given by

$$\omega(u) = \begin{cases} 0, & \text{if } 0 < u \leq 1, \\ \frac{1}{3}, & \text{if } 1 < u \leq 4, \\ 0, & \text{if } u > 3. \end{cases}$$

(a) Predict
  (i) the total size of the epidemic,
  (ii) the peak daily incidence attained during the epidemic,
  (iii) the duration of time from the introduction of the infectious disease to the time of peak incidence, and
  (iv) the duration of time the daily incidence is above 10.

(b) Suppose it is possible to immunize 20% of the community prior to the introduction of the infection. With such prior immunization in place make the same predictions as in part (a).

(c) Describe the extent to which such prior immunization mitigates the impact of the epidemic.

3. Using the data in Table 9.1, estimate the initial reproduction number R and the shape parameter α under the assumption that the probability distribution of the serial interval is given by probabilities

$$p_j = \begin{cases} 0, & \text{if } j = 1, 2, \ldots, 12, \\ \exp\left[-\left(\frac{j-13}{7}\right)^\alpha\right] - \exp\left[-\left(\frac{j-12}{7}\right)^\alpha\right], & \text{if } j = 13, 14, 15, \ldots . \end{cases}$$

Plot the graph of the p_j, using your estimated parameter values.

4. The age at infection is observed for a sample of cases in a community with endemic transmission of the infectious disease.

(a) Suppose the sample mean of the age at infection is 6.9 years, with standard error 0.2 years. Use the graph in Figure 9.9 to deduce a confidence interval for R_0.

(b) Suppose the sample mean of the age at infection is 16.9 years, with standard error 0.2 years. Deduce a confidence interval for R_0.

(c) Compare the confidence intervals found in (a) and (b). Propose a general conclusion about the way precision of the estimate of R_0 depends on age.

5. Consider a developing country that has had the same annual number of births for many years. Suppose each newly born individual has probability $q_j = \exp(-j\theta)$ of surviving to reach his, or her, j^{th} birthday and the mean life expectancy is 50 years. A certain infectious disease is endemic and the mean age at infection is 8 years.

   Estimate R_0, assuming that the only source of immunity is prior exposure to the disease.

6. A community consists of 1200 individuals of Type 1 and 800 individuals of Type 2. All are susceptible to a certain infectious disease. The median of the infectivity profile is 4 days, for both types of infective.
   Suppose one initial (newly infected) infective of Type 1 joins the community. The mean of the number of Type 1 individuals he infects is 0.6 and the mean of the number of Type 2 individuals he infects is 0.8.
   If, instead, the initial infective is of Type 2, the mean of the number of Type 1 individuals he infects is 1.2 and the mean of the number of Type 2 individuals he infects is 2.0.

   (a) Using generation time, produce the epidemic curves for
      (i) Type 1 infectives,
      (ii) Type 2 infectives, and
      (iii) the total infectives

      when an epidemic is initiated by one infective of Type 2.

   (b) Suppose 600 Type 1 individuals are vaccinated, with a fully protective vaccine, before one infective of Type 2 initiates an epidemic.
      Predict how much these prior vaccinations change
      (i) the maximum number of daily infections,
      (ii) the time taken to reach the peak of the epidemic.

   (c) Suppose now, instead, that 600 Type 2 individuals are vaccinated before one infective of Type 2 initiates an epidemic.
      Predict how much these prior vaccinations change
      (i) the maximum number of daily infections,
      (ii) the time taken to reach the peak of the epidemic

      for this selection of vaccinees.

   (d) Compare the benefit of prior vaccination for these two ways of selecting susceptibles for vaccination.

9.6 Supplementary material

9.6.1 Epidemic curve in incremental time steps

As in Section 9.1.1, we consider a uniformly mixing community of size $n+1$, where n is large. The community has been free from a certain infectious disease when one community member is infected by an external contact. This point in time is taken as the time origin and time is measured in days. It is assumed that an epidemic occurs and our aim is to describe the epidemic curve by a deterministic model.

Model equations for such a deterministic model are introduced in Section 8.10.1. It is not possible to obtain an explicit algebraic expression for the epidemic curve from these equations, so we describe how to compute the epidemic curve numerically with the aid of a computer. We do this by specifying, iteratively, the amount of transmission that occurs in each of the large number of small time increments $(0, \delta]$, $(\delta, 2\delta]$, $(2\delta, 3\delta]$, $\ldots$.

Let $S(t)$ denote the "number of susceptibles" remaining in the community at time t, i.e., t days after the introduction of the infectious disease into the community. In particular, $S(0)$ is the number of susceptibles in the community immediately after the introduction of the infectious disease into the community. Let $I(j\delta)$ denote the "number of new infections" arising during the period from time $(j-1)\delta$ to time $j\delta$, $j = 1, 2, 3, \ldots$.

If the basic reproduction number of our infectious disease is R_0 and the infectivity profile is $\omega(u)$, $u \geq 0$, we compute

$$I(\delta) \;=\; R_0\, \omega(0)\, I(0)\, \frac{S(0)}{n}\, \delta\,,$$

where $I(0) = 1$, corresponding to the initial infective, and $I(\delta)$ is the mean *amount* of infection generated by the initial infective over the first time increment. To get the amount of infection over $(\delta, 2\delta]$, the second time increment, we first adjust the remaining number of susceptibles to $S(\delta) = S(0) - I(\delta)$ and then compute

$$I(2\delta) \;=\; R_0 \left[\omega(0)\, I(\delta) + \omega(\delta)\, I(0)\right] \frac{S(\delta)}{n}\, \delta\,.$$

Corresponding to the third increment we compute $S(2\delta) = S(\delta) - I(\delta)$ and

$$I(3\delta) \;=\; R_0 \left[\omega(0)\, I(2\delta) + \omega(\delta)\, I(\delta) + \omega(2\delta)\, I(0)\right] \frac{S(2\delta)}{n}\, \delta\,.$$

In this way we compute the "number of new infections" for each successive interval until we reach the end of the epidemic.

Figure 9.1 shows an example of an epidemic curve computed in this way.

A modification that is more robust to the choice of time increments

It is tempting to steer away from small values of δ, to avoid lengthy computing times. However, for certain infectious disease characteristics, e.g. when R is large and the latent period is short, choosing a larger value for δ can lead to a poor approximation, including the possibility that the number of new infections in the next time increment exceeds the number of remaining susceptibles. To avoid the latter problem, it is safer to modify the above iterative equations a little. We illustrate the modification with respect to the third time increment.

Note that over the time increment $(2\delta, 3\delta]$, every remaining susceptible, independently, has probability

$$\exp\{-R_0\,[\omega(0)\,I(2\delta)+\omega(\delta)\,I(\delta)+\omega(2\delta)\,I(0)]\,\delta/n\}$$

of avoiding infection; see Section 5.6.2. Therefore, the mean number of the remaining susceptibles infected during the time increment $(2\delta, 3\delta]$ is

$$I(3\delta)=S(2\delta)\Big[1-\exp\{-R_0\,[\omega(0)\,I(2\delta)+\omega(\delta)\,I(\delta)+\omega(2\delta)\,I(0)]\,\delta/n\}\Big].$$

An analogous modification is made for other time increments. This approximation is less likely to lead to unrealistic extremes when the chosen value of δ is too large for the characteristics of the infectious disease.

9.6.2 Age at infection

The time A until a newborn individual is infected is called the age at infection. When the infection is endemic in the community the infection intensity acting on an individual is essentially a constant, λ say. It follows that the random variable A has an exponential distribution with probability density function

$$f(a) = \lambda\exp(-\lambda a), \quad a \geq 0,$$

because the negative exponential distribution is the distribution that corresponds to a constant hazard function. This gives the probability that an individual is not infected by age a as

$$\Pr(A > a) = \exp(-\lambda a).$$

The maximum likelihood estimate of λ from the observed age at the time of infection for n individuals is $\hat{\lambda} = 1/\bar{a}$, where $\bar{a}$ is the sample mean of a sample of observed ages at infection. The form of this maximum likelihood estimate seems natural when we recall that the mean of the exponential distribution is given by $\mathrm{E}(A) = 1/\lambda$.

9.7 Bibliographic notes

A comprehensive coverage of deterministic epidemic models is given in the classic book by Anderson and May (1991). Included are age-dependent transmission models, which permit discussion of the age at which a vaccine should be administered for the best control of an infectious disease.

A way to use incidence data for the estimation of the initial reproduction number, and to monitor the change in R over time, is described by Wallinga and Teunis (2004). The approach we described in Section 9.2 is proposed by White and Pagano (2008).

CHAPTER 10

Using data to inform model choice

Our focus has been on showing how specific infectious disease models can be used to gain insights into infectious disease control. The models are formulated to reflect how person-to-person transmission occurs and therefore seem plausible. However, we have deliberately kept models simple and it is possible that a crucial characteristic of the infection's transmission in our community is not captured by the proposed model. Whenever possible, we should check that descriptions provided by our model are in accordance with observed data.

This chapter discusses ways infectious disease data can be used to inform model choice. In the core of this chapter we illustrate the statistical detective work involved in finding a model that adequately describes infectious disease data on household outbreaks. Briefly, two sets of data on the size of household outbreaks of measles are compared and the difference between them is then explored by modifying features of a transmission model until a plausible explanation for the difference is found.

The models introduced in the core of this chapter are extended to larger households in Section 10.6.

10.1 Model-free comparison of data on outbreak size

Table 10.1: *Observed frequencies for the size of measles outbreaks in Cirencester and Providence households of size three*

Outbreak size	Cirencester	Providence
1	6	34
2	11	25
3	43	275
Total	60	334

Consider data on size of outbreak for measles in households having three susceptible members. Table 10.1 summarizes two such data sets that were presented by Bailey (1975), one from Cirencester in the UK, with 60 households, and the other from Providence, Rhode Island, with 334 households.

Each outbreak is started by one primary case, who contracted measles outside the household. The relative frequencies of different outbreak sizes displayed in Figure 10.1 provide a visual comparison of the two sets of outbreaks. The high relative frequencies for outbreak size 3 reflects the highly infectious nature of measles.

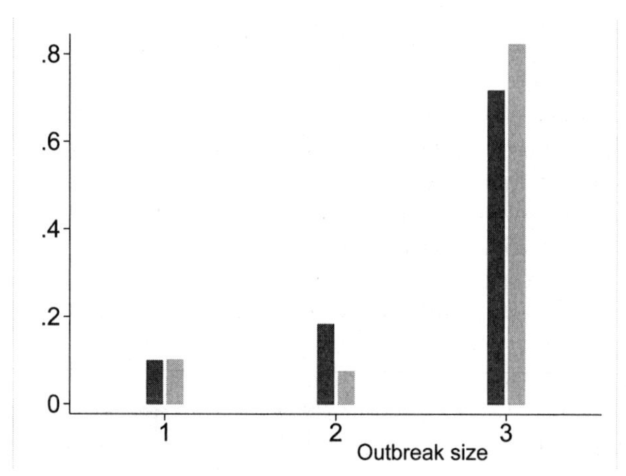

Figure 10.1 *Relative frequencies for measles outbreak sizes in households of three susceptibles observed in Cirencester (dark) and Providence, Rhode Island (light).*

Our primary aim might be to use these data to quantify the transmission rate of measles within households. For this purpose it would be useful to pool the information from the two data sets, because this usually gives a more precise estimate of the probability of transmission between household members. Before we can pool the data we must ensure that there is no evidence that the characteristics of measles transmission differ between the two locations. We begin by comparing outbreak size without making assumptions about disease transmission.

A general statistical model for data of the type in Table 10.1 is described by the following notation. For each household, let θ_j denote the probability that j of the three susceptibles become cases by the end of the outbreak. Data on n such outbreaks can be summarized by observations on N_1, N_2 and N_3, the number of households with exactly 1, 2 and 3 cases, respectively. The marginal distribution for N_j is the Binomial distribution, with n trials and success probability θ_j. The joint distribution of (N_1, N_2, N_3) is the trinomial distribution specified by

$$\Pr(N_1 = n_1, N_2 = n_2, N_3 = n_3) = \frac{n!}{n_1!\, n_2!\, n_3!}\, \theta_1^{n_1} \theta_2^{n_2} \theta_3^{n_3},$$

where $n_1 + n_2 + n_3 = n$ and $\theta_1 + \theta_2 + \theta_3 = 1$.

The form of this distribution applies to both Cirencester and Providence, but the value of n differs in the two locations and the probabilities θ_1, θ_2 and θ_3 might also differ. We wish to test whether the distributions for the two locations have the same values of θ_1, θ_2 and θ_3. Under the null hypothesis that the probability distribution of outbreak size is the same in the two locations, the likelihood function corresponding to the data in Table 10.1 is

$$\ell(\theta_1, \theta_2) = c \times \theta_1^{6+34} \theta_2^{11+25} \theta_3^{43+275} = c \times \theta_1^{40} \theta_2^{36} (1 - \theta_1 + \theta_2)^{318},$$

where c is a constant. The maximum likelihood estimates are given by $\hat{\theta}_1 = 40/394$, $\hat{\theta}_2 = 36/394$ and $\hat{\theta}_3 = 1 - \hat{\theta}_1 - \hat{\theta}_2 = 318/394$.

Table 10.2 shows the expected frequencies $\mathrm{E}(N_j) = n\theta_j$, the observed frequencies and the fitted frequencies $n\hat{\theta}_j$, where $n = 60$ for Cirencester and $n = 334$ for Providence.

Table 10.2: *Observed and fitted frequencies for household outbreak sizes of measles in Cirencester and Providence*

		Cirencester		Providence	
Outbreak size	Expected	Observed	Fitted	Observed	Fitted
1	$n\theta_1$	6	6.1	34	33.9
2	$n\theta_2$	11	5.5	25	30.5
3	$n\theta_3$	43	48.4	275	269.6

The goodness-of-fit statistic for testing the null hypothesis that the distribution of outbreak size is the same for the two locations is

$$\sum \frac{(n_j - n\hat{\theta}_j)^2}{n\hat{\theta}_j} = \frac{(6 - 6.1)^2}{6.1} + \cdots + \frac{(275 - 269.6)^2}{269.6} = 7.3,$$

where the summation is over the six observed frequencies. Comparing the realized value of the test statistic with percentiles of the χ_2^2-distribution, the chi-squared distribution with two degrees of freedom, gives a p-value of 0.026. At the 5% level of significance there is evidence that the distribution of outbreak size differs for the two locations.

While we explained the above analysis in terms of maximum likelihood estimation of parameters, the easiest way to implement it is to feed the six observed frequencies into a statistical computer package and perform an analysis for a 3×2 contingency table. This computer analysis is equivalent to the one described above.

It is of interest to explore plausible reasons for the difference in the two distributions of outbreak size of Table 10.1 and that is the main theme of Sections 10.2 and 10.3. To find a plausible reason for the difference we look for a transmission model that adequately describes each data set, beginning with the simplest type of model.

10.2 Transmission among homogeneous individuals

Assume that one of the three susceptible household members acquires infection from a contact outside the household and thereafter the household outbreak evolves without further community-acquired transmission. Also assume that individuals are homogeneous, with regard to susceptibility and infectivity, and that household members mix uniformly with each other. We formulate a transmission model for the size of outbreaks of measles in such a setting, as an alternative to the trinomial model used in Section 10.1.

10.2.1 A transmission model for outbreak size

To transform the general trinomial model into a transmission model, we need to express the parameters θ_1, θ_2 and θ_3 in terms of epidemiological parameters that quantify the chance that the infection passes from one person to another.

Consider first the parameter θ_1, the probability that the outbreak size is 1. The outbreak size can be 1 only if each of the two initial susceptibles avoids infection by the primary household infective. We assume that they are exposed to the primary infective independently. Then $\theta_1 = q^2$, where q is the probability that a given susceptible avoids infection by one infective member of the same household when exposed for the entire duration of the infectious period. The probability expression $\theta_1 = q^2$ relies on three assumptions mentioned above, namely the independence, the homogeneity of the susceptibles and that infection from outside the household is negligible when compared with transmission within the household once the infection has been introduced into the household.

The outbreak is of size 2 if the primary infective infects exactly one of the initial susceptibles and the remaining susceptible also avoids infection by the secondary case. The probability of this outcome is $2q(1-q) \times q$, again using the assumptions of independence and homogeneity. The probability that all three individuals are eventually cases is determined by the probabilities summing to 1. This gives the probability distribution shown in Table 10.3, where the notation $\tilde{q} = 1 - q$ is used for convenience.

Table 10.3: *Outbreak size model assuming homogeneity*

		Observed frequency	
Outbreak size	Probability	Cirencester	Providence
1	q^2	6	34
2	$2\tilde{q}q^2$	11	25
3	$\tilde{q}^2(1+2q)$	43	275

In summary, this transmission model expresses the parameters θ_1, θ_2

and θ_3 in terms of the single parameter q, the probability that a given susceptible avoids infection by one infective member of the same household when exposed for the entire duration of the infectious period.

Consider now if the data on outbreak size observed for Cirencester and Providence can be described adequately by this model. The same form of model might describe each data set, but with a different value for the parameter q. We estimate the parameter of the model from the observed frequencies by the method of maximum likelihood. For example, the likelihood function corresponding to the Cirencester data is given by

$$\ell(q) = \text{constant} \times (q^2)^6(\tilde{q}q^2)^{11}[\tilde{q}^2(1+2q)]^{43}, \qquad 0 \leq q \leq 1.$$

There is no explicit expression for the maximum likelihood estimate of q, so a numerical method is needed to find the value of q that maximizes the likelihood $\ell(q)$. This can be done by using a spreadsheet or by using statistical computer software.

The constraint $0 \leq q \leq 1$ may cause difficulties when statistical computer software is used to obtain the maximum likelihood estimate. This can be overcome by rewriting the model in terms of a parameter that is not constrained. One such parameter is

$$\varphi = \ln\left(\frac{q}{1-q}\right), \quad \text{which may be solved to give} \quad q = \frac{\exp(\varphi)}{1+\exp(\varphi)}.$$

For the Cirencester data this gives the maximum likelihood estimate of q to be $\hat{q}_{\text{C}} = 0.347$.

Similarly we obtain the maximum likelihood estimate of q for the Providence data to be $\hat{q}_{\text{RI}} = 0.272$. Substituting these estimates into the probability expressions for our model and multiplying by the total number of outbreaks, for each locality, gives the fitted frequencies shown in Table 10.4.

Table 10.4: *Fitted frequencies when we assume homogeneity*

		Cirencester		Providence	
Outbreak size	Expected	Observed	Fitted	Observed	Fitted
1	nq^2	6	7.2	34	24.7
2	$2n\tilde{q}q^2$	11	9.5	25	36.0
3	$n\tilde{q}^2(1+2q)$	43	43.3	275	273.3

The goodness-of-fit statistic for testing the concordance of the observed and fitted frequencies is 0.47 on one degree of freedom for Cirencester, giving a p-value of 0.49. This indicates that a transmission model based on the assumption that individuals are homogeneous and mix uniformly within households is a plausible description of the Cirencester data. For Providence the test statistics is 6.85 on one degree of freedom, giving a p-value of 0.009. Clearly this is not a satisfactory fit.

We conclude that, for the Providence data, there is an essential characteristic missing in the model. Further analysis is required to find a plausible description of the transmission process in households of Providence.

There is limited scope for further analysis when the data consist only of observed counts for three compartments. Fortunately the observed data on the outbreaks in Providence households are a little more detailed. To describe the enhanced data set we revisit the notion of a chain of transmission, which we introduced in Section 2.7.1.

10.2.2 Chains of transmission

As the name suggests, a chain of transmission contains some information about the progress of transmission among susceptibles of the household. Consider the introduction of an infectious disease into a household and assume that the risk of further infections from external contacts over the duration of the household outbreak is negligible compared with the risk of being infected by an internal household contact. In other words, after the introduction, the household outbreak essentially evolves in isolation.

The introductory, or primary, household infectives are cases of Generation 1. Generation 2 consists of cases who are not introductory cases, but had at least one direct infectious contact with an introductory case. All individuals who avoided infection by introductory cases, but made at least one direct infectious contact with an infective from Generation 2, make up Generation 3, and so on.

A transmission chain for an affected household is the enumeration of the number of cases in each generation, including Generation 1. For example, for a household with at least 4 members, we write $1 \rightarrow 1 \rightarrow 2$ to denote the chain consisting of one introductory case, one second generation case, two third generation cases and no cases in the fourth, or later, generations. It is notationally convenient to list only generations that contain cases. Therefore, a chain written $I_1 \rightarrow I_2 \rightarrow \cdots \rightarrow I_r$ will have $I_r > 0$ and implies that $I_{r+1} = 0$.

For outbreaks in households of size three, initiated by one introductory case, the possible transmission chains are 1, $1 \rightarrow 1$, $1 \rightarrow 1 \rightarrow 1$ and $1 \rightarrow 2$. The assumption that individuals are exposed to the primary infective independently implies that the probability of observing Chain 1 is q^2. Similarly we obtain the remaining expressions for chain probabilities shown in column three of Table 10.5, where $\tilde{q} = 1 - q$.

The outbreak sizes corresponding to transmission chains 1, $1 \rightarrow 1$, $1 \rightarrow 1 \rightarrow 1$ and $1 \rightarrow 2$ are 1, 2, 3 and 3, respectively. Therefore the probability distribution for outbreak size is easily deduced from Table 10.5 and is seen to agree with the distribution given in Table 10.3, as it should.

The transmission chains corresponding to the household outbreaks in Providence were identified and frequencies for the different chains are given

Table 10.5: *Fitted transmission chain model assuming homogeneity*

			Frequency		
Chain	Outbreak size	Probability	Expected	Observed	Fitted
1	1	q^2	nq^2	34	14.9
1→1	2	$2\tilde{q}q^2$	$2n\tilde{q}q^2$	25	23.5
1→1→1	3	$2\tilde{q}^2q$	$2n\tilde{q}^2q$	36	87.8
1→2	3	$\tilde{q}^2$	$n\tilde{q}^2$	239	207.8

in column five of Table 10.5. The transmission chain model is not expected to describe the observed chain frequencies adequately, since the observed outbreak size frequencies differ significantly from frequencies expected under these model assumptions. We will nevertheless fit the transmission chain model to the data, primarily to show that for the chain data the likelihood has a simple form and maximum likelihood estimation is straightforward.

The likelihood function corresponding to the Providence chain frequencies is given by

$$\ell(q) = c \times (q^2)^{34}(\tilde{q}q^2)^{25}(\tilde{q}^2q)^{36}(\tilde{q}^2)^{239} = c \times q^{154}(1-q)^{575}, \quad 0 \leq q \leq 1.$$

Note that the likelihood function has a form as for a Binomial distribution, allowing us to deduce that the maximum likelihood estimate of q is given by $\hat{q} = 154/(154+575)$. Substituting $n = 334$ and $q = \hat{q}$ into the expressions for the expected frequencies gives the fitted frequencies of Table 10.5. As expected, the fitted frequencies are not close to the observed frequencies.

We now explore modifications to the assumptions of the transmission chain model that might lead to an adequate description of the observed transmission chain data of Table 10.5.

10.3 Allowing transmission rates to differ between individuals

What is the missing ingredient in the above transmission model for the Providence data? It might be that the assumption of homogeneity of individuals is not appropriate, so let's allow individuals to differ. Individuals can differ by overt factors, such as gender or age, or by factors that are more difficult to observe, perhaps the condition of their immune system or behavioral characteristics. The Providence data set does not contain additional information on individuals and so we need to allow for heterogeneity in a way that does not require additional data.

Suppose the probability of disease transmission differs between pairs of individuals. Label the primary infective A and the other two individuals B and C. Let Q_{AB} denote the probability that individual B avoids having an infectious contact with primary infective A. If B is infected, let Q_{BC} denote the probability that individual C avoids having an infectious contact with the secondary infective B. Define Q_{AC} and Q_{CB} similarly. Then using the assumption that individuals are exposed to infectives independently we can deduce the chain transmission probabilities shown in Table 10.6, where $\tilde{x}$ denotes $1 - x$ for any variable x.

Table 10.6: *Transmission chain model with heterogeneity*

Chain	Conditional probability
1	$Q_{AB}\, Q_{AC}$
1→1	$\widetilde{Q}_{AB}\, Q_{AC}\, Q_{BC} + \widetilde{Q}_{AC}\, Q_{AB}\, Q_{CB}$
1→1→1	$\widetilde{Q}_{AB}\, Q_{AC}\, \widetilde{Q}_{BC} + \widetilde{Q}_{AC}\, Q_{AB}\, \widetilde{Q}_{CB}$
1→2	$\widetilde{Q}_{AB}\, \widetilde{Q}_{AC}$

The chain probabilities in Table 10.6 are conditional probabilities, given the values of Q_{AB}, Q_{AC}, Q_{BC} and Q_{CB}, which may be distinct for each pair of individuals. The chain probabilities reduce to those given in Table 10.5 when $Q_{AB} = Q_{AC} = Q_{BC} = Q_{CB} = q$, as they should. Alternative relationships between the Q's of Table 10.6 can reflect differences between individuals or different relationships between pairs. We use this idea to look for a plausible description of the Providence transmission chain data.

10.3.1 Variable infectivity

One possible explanation for the inadequate fit found in Table 10.5 is that individuals differ in how infectious they are. For example, infected individuals might differ in the duration of their infectious period, in the extent to which they shed pathogen or in the way they adjust their mixing behavior upon show of symptoms.

Suppose that individuals differ only in infectivity. We may then write $Q_{AB} = Q_{AC} = Q_A$, $Q_{BC} = Q_B$ and $Q_{CB} = Q_C$, giving the chain probabilities shown in column two of Table 10.7. This distribution for the transmission chains has one parameter corresponding to each individual of the household, and the same holds for every other household. No statistical inference is possible when we allow all of these Q's to be distinct parameters. Instead, we accommodate this kind of heterogeneity by considering each Q_A, Q_B and Q_C, in every household, to be an independent realization of a common random variable. This is a standard statistical approach for dealing with problems that arise from having too many parameters. It means that the probabilities in column two of Table 10.7 are conditional probabilities, given the values of Q_A, Q_B and Q_C. To obtain the unconditional probabilities we take the expectation of each probability in column two. In doing so we assume that Q_A, Q_B and Q_C are independent random variables with the same mean q and the same standard deviation σ. This leads to the chain probability model shown in the final column of Table 10.7. In this way we reduce the number of parameters to two, namely q and σ. Again, $\tilde{q}$ is used to denote $1 - q$ and a similar notation is used for other quantities. Note that these chain probabilities reduce to those of Table 10.5 when $\sigma = 0$, which corresponds to homogeneous infectivity.

Table 10.7: *Transmission chain model when infectivity differs*

Chain	Conditional probability	Unconditional probability
1	Q_A^2	$q^2 + \sigma^2$
1→1	$\widetilde{Q}_A\, Q_A\, (Q_B + Q_C)$	$2q(\tilde{q}q - \sigma^2)$
1→1→1	$\widetilde{Q}_A\, Q_A\, (\widetilde{Q}_B + \widetilde{Q}_C)$	$2\tilde{q}(\tilde{q}q - \sigma^2)$
1→2	$\widetilde{Q}_A^2$	$\tilde{q}^2 + \sigma^2$

The likelihood function corresponding to the Providence chain frequencies for the model of Table 10.7 is given by

$$\ell(q, \sigma) = \text{constant} \times (q^2 + \sigma^2)^{34} (\tilde{q}q^2 - q\sigma^2)^{25} (\tilde{q}^2 q - \tilde{q}\sigma^2)^{36} (\tilde{q}^2 + \sigma^2)^{239},$$

with $0 \leq q \leq 1$ and $\sigma > 0$. This likelihood function is maximized by the values $\hat{q} = 0.218$ and $\hat{\sigma} = 0.271$. Substituting these estimates and $n = 334$ into the expected frequencies gives the fitted frequencies shown in the final column of Table 10.8. Comparing the fitted frequencies with the observed frequencies clearly reveals that this model does not describe the data adequately. Formally, the goodness-of-fit statistic has the value 14.1, with one degree of freedom, giving a p-value less than 0.001. There is strong evidence that the model, with heterogeneity in infectivity, does not describe the data adequately.

Table 10.8: *Fitted chain model when infectivity differs*

Chain	Expected	Observed	Fitted
1	$n(q^2 + \sigma^2)$	34	40.5
1→1	$2nq(\tilde{q}q - \sigma^2)$	25	14.1
1→1→1	$2n\tilde{q}(\tilde{q}q - \sigma^2)$	36	50.7
1→2	$n(\tilde{q}^2 + \sigma^2)$	239	228.7

We need to try another kind of modification to the transmission model.

10.3.2 Variable susceptibility

Suppose now that susceptibility varies between individuals, while infectivity does not. Returning to the probabilities in Table 10.6, we now write $Q_{AB} = Q_{CB} = Q_B$ and $Q_{AC} = Q_{BC} = Q_C$, giving the chain probabilities shown in column two of Table 10.9. They are conditional probabilities, given Q_B and Q_C. We obtain the unconditional probabilities by assuming that Q_B and Q_C are independent random variables with the same mean q and the same standard deviation σ. Taking expectations of the conditional probabilities gives the probability model shown in column three of Table 10.9. Note that the interpretation of σ here differs from that in Table 10.7 and Table 10.8. Specifically, σ now reflects variation in the susceptibility of individuals, rather than variation in infectivity.

Table 10.9: *Transmission chain model when susceptibility differs*

Chain	Conditional probability	Unconditional probability
1	$Q_B\,Q_C$	q^2
1→1	$\tilde{Q}_B\,Q_C^2 + \tilde{Q}_C\,Q_B^2$	$2\tilde{q}(q^2+\sigma^2)$
1→1→1	$\tilde{Q}_B\,Q_C\,\tilde{Q}_C + \tilde{Q}_C\,Q_B\,\tilde{Q}_B$	$2\tilde{q}(\tilde{q}q-\sigma^2)$
1→2	$\tilde{Q}_B\,\tilde{Q}_C$	$\tilde{q}^2$

The maximum likelihood estimates of q and σ for the Providence data are obtained by maximizing the likelihood function

$$\ell(q,\sigma) = \text{constant} \times (q^2)^{34}(\tilde{q}q^2+\tilde{q}\sigma^2)^{25}(\tilde{q}^2q-\tilde{q}\sigma^2)^{36}(\tilde{q}^2)^{239}$$

with respect to q and σ. This gives the estimates $\hat{q}=0.193$ and $\hat{\sigma}=0.205$, which leads to the fitted frequencies shown in the final column of Table 10.10.

Table 10.10: *Fitted model when susceptibility differs*

Chain	Expected	Observed	Fitted
1	nq^2	34	12.5
1→1	$2n\tilde{q}(q^2+\sigma^2)$	25	42.7
1→1→1	$2n\tilde{q}(\tilde{q}q-\sigma^2)$	36	61.4
1→2	$n\tilde{q}^2$	239	217.5

A comparison of the observed and fitted frequencies clearly indicates that this model also fails to give an adequate fit to the data. Formally, the goodness-of-fit statistic has the value 57.2, with one degree of freedom, giving a p-value much less than 0.001. There is very strong evidence that heterogeneity in susceptibility, as modeled here, does not give a satisfactory description of these data.

We need to try yet another kind of modification to the transmission model.

10.3.3 *Variable households*

Instead of looking for heterogeneity among all individuals let us allow households to differ, but leave individuals within any one household homogeneous. It may be that different levels of hygiene or different levels of crowding are an essential feature of transmission of measles in households.

Returning to the conditional probabilities given in Table 10.6, we set $Q_{AB} = Q_{AC} = Q_{BC} = Q_{CB} = Q$. This gives a model like the simple model in column three of Table 10.5. However, to allow for heterogeneity among households, we take Q to be a random variable. In other words, Q may have a different value for each household. Taking expectations of the conditional chain probabilities, given in column two of Table 10.11, introduces three characteristics of the distribution of Q, namely $\mathrm{E}(Q)$, $\mathrm{E}(Q^2)$ and $\mathrm{E}(Q^3)$.

Table 10.11: *Transmission chain model when households differs*

Chain	Conditional probability	Unconditional probability
1	Q^2	$q^2 + \sigma^2$
1→1	$2\tilde{Q}\,Q^2$	$2\tilde{q}(q^2 + \sigma^2)(\tilde{q}q - \sigma^2)/(\tilde{q}q + \sigma^2)$
1→1→1	$2\tilde{Q}^2 Q$	$2q(\tilde{q}^2 + \sigma^2)(\tilde{q}q - \sigma^2)/(\tilde{q}q + \sigma^2)$
1→2	$\tilde{Q}^2$	$\tilde{q}^2 + \sigma^2$

Without restricting the family of distributions for Q, three parameters are needed to specify the unconditional chain probabilities. This is really too many parameters when we have data on only four frequencies (with three degrees of freedom). We therefore assume that Q has a Beta distribution, given by density function

$$f(x) = \text{constant} \times x^{a-1}(1-x)^{b-1}, \qquad 0 < x < 1,$$

where the constant is such that the area under the density function f is equal to 1. The parameters a and b may have any positive value. They need to be estimated from the chain frequency data. Assuming that Q has a Beta distribution is a minimal constraint, as this is a diverse family of distributions. Taking expectations of the conditional chain probabilities under this assumption gives the unconditional probabilities in column three of Table 10.11, in terms of the two parameters $q = \mathrm{E}(Q)$ and $\sigma^2 = \mathrm{Var}(Q)$. The parameters q and σ^2 are used because they have a more direct epidemiological interpretation than do a and b. Specifically, σ now reflects variation in the transmission probability between households.

The maximum likelihood estimates of q and σ, corresponding to the Providence data, are $\hat{q} = 0.195$ and $\hat{\sigma} = 0.258$. They give the fitted frequencies shown in the final column of Table 10.12 and are seen to be in excellent agreement with the observed frequencies. Specifically, the value of the chi-square goodness-of-fit criterion for this fitted model is 0.3, with one degree of freedom, corresponding to a p-value of 0.57.

Table 10.12: *Fitted transmission chain model when households differ*

Chain	Expected	Observed	Fitted
1	$n(q^2+\sigma^2)$	34	34.9
1→1	$2n\tilde{q}(q^2+\sigma^2)(\tilde{q}q-\sigma^2)/(\tilde{q}q+\sigma^2)$	25	22.7
1→1→1	$2nq(\tilde{q}^2+\sigma^2)(\tilde{q}q-\sigma^2)/(\tilde{q}q+\sigma^2)$	36	37.6
1→2	$n(\tilde{q}^2+\sigma^2)$	239	238.8

We conclude that variability among households in Providence is a plausible explanation of the observed difference between household outbreaks of measles in Cirencester and Providence.

10.4 Discussion

Our analysis of the Cirencester data on size of measles outbreaks suggests that measles transmission in Cirencester can be described in terms of individuals who are homogeneous across households and mix similarly within households. In contrast, there is significant evidence to suggest that transmission among homogeneous individuals who mix similarly within households does not describe measles transmission in Providence. The missing characteristic of measles transmission in Providence is unlikely to be independent variation in infectivity or independent variation in susceptibility, but it could be that the within-household transmission probabilities vary between households. Such variation might stem from variation in the level of crowding or hygiene in the households of Providence.

Our analysis is based largely on goodness-of-fit tests for models. When interpreting results, it is therefore important to remember the difference between accepting a null hypothesis and rejecting a null hypothesis. The null hypothesis is always given "the benefit of doubt" and so accepting the "adequacy-of-fit" of a model is not a strong endorsement of the model. On the other hand, rejecting the "adequacy-of-fit" indicates substantial evidence that an essential model component is missing. Thus the adequacy of the models in Table 10.3 and Table 10.11 for the Cirencester and Providence data, respectively, provides plausible descriptions, but there may be other models that also provide plausible descriptions, some of which are explored in Exercise 1 of Section 10.5.

Our strongest results are those that reject the "adequacy-of-fit" to the Providence data. Specifically, we have learnt that some heterogeneity among individuals must be allowed for to adequately describe the Providence data, and that neither independent variation in infectivity among individuals nor independent variation in susceptibility among individuals is the right kind of heterogeneity.

10.5 Exercises

1. The Cirencester household outbreaks of measles were also classified into transmission chains, with observed chain frequencies given by

Chain	1	1→1	1→1→1	1→2
Frequency	6	11	6	37

   (a) Use the method of maximum likelihood to obtain parameter estimates for the transmission chain model with

      (i) homogeneous individuals who mix uniformly, as in Table 10.5,
      (ii) variable infectivity, as in Table 10.7,
      (iii) variable susceptibility, as in Table 10.9, and
      (iv) variation among households, as in Table 10.11.

   (b) In each case compute the fitted frequencies, perform the goodness-of-fit test and state your conclusions.

2. Consider a household with five susceptible members and suppose that two of them are infected, simultaneously, by an outside contact. In other words, the household outbreak begins with two primary infectives and three initial susceptibles. For this household outbreak

   (a) enumerate the possible transmission chains, and
   (b) determine the probability for each chain, using the chain-binomial assumption.

3. The possible transmission chains for a household outbreak initiated by one infective with four susceptible household partners are given in Table 10.13, together with the probabilities of these chains under the chain-binomial model introduced in Section 10.6; see column two of Table 10.17. The interpretation of the model parameters is as follows:

   q is the probability that a susceptible avoids ever being infected when exposed to one specific infective,

   q_2 is the probability that a susceptible avoids ever being infected when exposed to two specific infectives, and

   q_3 is the probability that a susceptible avoids ever being infected when exposed to three specific infectives.

   Also given in Table 10.13 are the observed frequencies of these chains among 664 such household outbreaks of the common cold, as presented by Heasman and Reid (1961).

Table 10.13: *Frequencies for transmission chains of the common cold in households with five susceptibles*

Chain	Chain probability	Observed frequency
1	q^4	423
1→1	$4q^6(1-q)$	131
1→1→1	$12q^7(1-q)^2$	36
1→2	$6q^2(1-q)^2q_2^2$	24
1→1→1→1	$24q^7(1-q)^3$	14
1→1→2	$12q^4(1-q)^3q_2$	8
1→2→1	$12q^3(1-q)^2q_2(1-q_2)$	11
1→3	$4q(1-q)^3q_3$	3
1→1→1→1→1	$24q^6(1-q)^4$	4
1→1→1→2	$12q^5(1-q)^4$	2
1→1→2→1	$12q^4(1-q)^3(1-q_2)$	2
1→1→3	$4q^3(1-q)^4$	2
1→2→1→1	$12q^2(1-q)^3q_2(1-q_2)$	3
1→2→2	$6q^2(1-q)^2(1-q_2)^2$	1
1→3→1	$4q(1-q)^3(1-q_3)$	0
1→4	$(1-q)^4$	0
Total	1	664

(a) Discuss difficulties that would be encountered in identifying the transmission chains for household outbreaks of the common cold.

(b) Compute the maximum likelihood estimates of the parameters q, q_2 and q_3.

(c) Compute the "fitted frequencies," using estimates of q, q_2 and q_3.

(d) Compare the fitted and observed frequencies for the transmission chains by a goodness-of-fit test, or otherwise, to judge whether the model provides an adequate fit to the frequency counts.

(e) Does the Greenwood model, for which $q = q_2 = q_3$, provide an adequate fit to the frequency count data?

(f) Does the Reed-Frost model, for which $q_2 = q^2$ and $q_3 = q^3$, provide an adequate description of the frequency counts?

4. The household outbreaks of the common cold shown in Table 10.13 were classified according to the level of crowding in the household. This classification is given by:

Outbreak size	Frequency Overcrowded	Crowded	Uncrowded	Total
1	112	155	156	423
2	35	41	55	131
3	17	24	19	60
4	11	15	10	36
5	6	6	2	14
Total	181	241	242	664

Test the hypothesis that the distribution of outbreak size is the same for each level of crowding.

5. Table 10.14, on pages 184-187, summarizes some of the data collected when the entire measles epidemic in the village of Hagelloch was monitored daily in November and December of 1861. Virtually all susceptible children were infected. The variables are defined as follows:

PN = patient number	SEX (0 = unknown, 1 = male, 2 = female)
FN = family name	PRO = day of prodrome
HN = house number	ERU = day of onset of rash
AGE = age in years	CL = school attendance status (0 = preschool, 1 = class 1, 2 = class 2)

[Day 1 is October 30, 1861. Family name is given as a number. More than one family lived in some houses. A prodrome is an early symptom, such as fever, indicating onset of illness.]

Use the data to explore what characteristics should be included in a model to describe the dynamics of this measles epidemic.

Specifically, do the data contain evidence of

(a) different rates of transmission between males and females

  (i) within households?
  (ii) outside households?

(b) different rates of transmission between preschool children, class 1 children and class 2 children

  (i) within households?
  (ii) outside households?

Table 10.14: *Data from the Hagelloch measles epidemic*

PN	FN	HN	AGE	SEX	PRO	ERU	CL	PN	FN	HN	AGE	SEX	PRO	ERU	CL
1	41	61	7	2	23	27	1	25	35	46	12	2	32	36	2
2	41	61	6	2	25	29	1	26	67	78	7	1	24	29	1
3	41	61	4	2	30	34	0	27	29	31	5	1	32	34	0
4	61	62	13	1	29	30	2	28	65	74	10	2	27	32	2
5	42	63	8	2	24	29	1	29	15	2	13	1	32	34	2
6	42	63	12	1	28	31	2	30	15	2	11	2	27	31	2
7	26	23	6	1	26	30	0	31	15	2	9	2	23	26	1
8	44	69	10	1	23	28	1	32	15	2	7	1	23	26	1
9	44	69	13	1	28	32	2	33	1	2	7	2	26	28	1
10	29	31	7	2	23	27	1	34	1	2	11	1	23	28	2
11	27	25	11	2	27	32	2	35	10	38	13	2	27	32	2
12	32	44	7	2	22	27	1	36	46	20	11	1	33	37	2
13	32	44	13	1	32	37	2	37	46	20	13	1	27	34	2
14	22	16	13	2	24	31	2	38	54	20	12	0	31	37	2
15	22	16	8	1	26	31	1	39	5	11	10	1	25	28	1
16	43	65	15	2	23	27	2	40	36	47	13	1	35	39	2
17	43	65	10	2	22	27	2	41	59	41	12	1	29	31	2
18	43	65	2	2	25	29	0	42	33	45	4	2	17	21	0
19	11	46	11	1	22	26	2	43	33	45	2	1	28	32	0
20	11	46	10	1	24	29	2	44	45	80	10	1	24	26	1
21	11	46	13	2	25	31	2	45	48	51	7	1	13	15	1
22	35	46	10	2	23	27	1	46	48	51	13	1	23	29	2
23	35	46	7	2	23	27	1	47	48	51	11	2	26	29	2
24	35	46	4	1	32	36	0	48	29	31	3	2	33	37	0

Table 10.14 *(Continued)*

PN	FN	HN	AGE	SEX	PRO	ERU	CL	PN	FN	HN	AGE	SEX	PRO	ERU	CL
49	49	64	10	1	30	38	2	73	47	42	11	2	29	37	2
50	44	69	6	2	34	38	0	74	23	18	10	2	23	28	1
51	15	2	4	1	33	37	0	75	23	18	13	1	31	37	2
52	43	65	13	1	31	37	2	76	42	63	2	1	35	38	0
53	43	65	6	1	32	36	0	77	18	8	8	2	29	29	1
54	43	65	4	1	34	37	0	78	18	8	11	2	24	28	2
55	43	65	11	2	33	37	2	79	18	8	5	2	29	37	0
56	20	14	8	1	24	31	1	80	18	8	12	1	32	37	2
57	20	14	3	1	33	37	0	81	5	11	12	1	33	36	2
58	24	19	9	1	24	28	1	82	21	15	8	1	24	28	1
59	24	19	10	2	32	36	2	83	21	15	10	2	33	37	2
60	24	19	2	1	34	38	0	84	21	15	6	1	32	36	0
61	8	28	5	2	33	35	0	85	45	80	5	2	34	37	0
62	8	28	14	1	34	38	2	86	41	61	3	2	35	37	0
63	8	28	12	1	31	40	2	87	60	50	12	2	34	39	2
64	30	32	7	1	23	29	1	88	60	50	10	2	34	39	2
65	30	32	2	1	33	38	0	89	32	44	3	2	34	37	0
66	30	32	5	2	35	37	0	90	36	47	11	1	34	37	2
67	55	26	11	2	34	39	2	91	36	47	4	2	35	37	0
68	16	5	2	2	32	34	0	92	36	47	2	2	36	39	0
69	63	67	1	1	45	49	0	93	36	47	8	1	24	28	1
70	21	15	13	1	30	35	2	94	10	38	4	2	22	35	0
71	29	31	10	2	33	37	2	95	29	31	1.25	1	36	39	0
72	32	44	10	2	33	38	2	96	28	27	2	1	32	36	0

Table 10.14 *(Continued)*

PN	FN	HN	AGE	SEX	PRO	ERU	CL	PN	FN	HN	AGE	SEX	PRO	ERU	CL
97	28	27	10	1	23	27	1	121	50	24	10	1	38	40	2
98	27	25	3	1	33	44	0	122	50	24	1	2	37	42	0
99	27	25	5	1	36	42	0	123	25	22	1.5	2	35	39	0
100	69	24	12	1	35	39	2	124	7	21	3	1	37	40	0
101	26	23	7.5	2	36	38	0	125	7	21	2	2	39	41	0
102	68	79	12	1	35	39	2	126	54	20	5	0	37	41	0
103	54	20	12	0	35	39	2	127	34	45	1	1	39	41	0
104	24	19	5	1	36	38	0	128	6	12	5	1	35	37	0
105	23	18	3	1	37	40	0	129	6	12	4	2	37	39	0
106	34	45	4	1	25	28	0	130	20	14	12	2	32	38	2
107	34	45	12	2	32	39	2	131	20	14	1	1	37	38	0
108	34	45	6	1	36	38	0	132	22	16	11	1	35	39	2
109	32	44	6	2	37	39	0	133	53	17	2	2	37	40	0
110	49	64	3	1	36	38	0	134	18	8	13	1	33	38	2
111	2	3	12	1	33	37	2	135	18	8	2	1	38	39	0
112	2	3	10	1	35	40	2	136	12	69	13	2	31	39	2
113	15	2	0.5	2	36	39	0	137	12	69	10	2	33	38	2
114	52	7	13	0	33	37	2	138	3	4	11	0	33	37	2
115	66	77	11	2	33	39	2	139	3	4	13	0	39	43	2
116	40	60	8	1	23	27	1	140	58	37	2	0	37	42	0
117	40	60	14	1	34	38	2	141	50	24	4	2	87	90	0
118	40	60	2	2	34	38	0	142	39	59	5	1	37	40	0
119	40	60	0.5	2	33	40	0	143	39	59	11	2	37	40	2
120	26	23	1	1	38	40	0	144	39	59	2	1	38	40	0

Table 10.14 *(Continued)*

PN	FN	HN	AGE	SEX	PRO	ERU	CL	PN	FN	HN	AGE	SEX	PRO	ERU	CL
145	39	59	8	2	25	29	1	169	38	48	4	1	36	39	0
146	13	70	4	2	33	39	0	170	38	48	10	1	39	42	2
147	13	70	0.75	2	35	39	0	171	38	48	0.75	1	47	49	0
148	19	13	13	2	35	39	2	172	62	66	3	2	21	23	0
149	19	13	4	1	37	41	0	173	9	35	6	1	3	5	0
150	19	13	0.5	1	43	47	0	174	9	35	3	2	10	10	0
151	37	48	2	2	39	43	0	175	9	35	2	1	14	17	0
152	37	48	4	2	38	40	0	176	64	70	0.5	0	43	47	0
153	37	48	10	2	26	29	1	177	17	6	8	2	9	13	1
154	37	48	6	2	35	36	0	178	17	6	4	1	9	13	0
155	47	42	13	1	41	45	2	179	17	6	1	2	20	23	1
156	31	42	8	1	24	26	1	180	17	6	10	1	19	23	2
157	31	42	4	2	36	39	0	181	4	6	10	2	15	19	2
158	31	42	3	2	36	39	0	182	4	6	13	1	17	20	2
159	46	20	2	2	41	45	0	183	4	6	4	1	13	17	0
160	16	5	0.5	2	44	45	0	184	51	6	13	0	1	8	2
161	19	13	6	2	44	48	0	185	21	15	3	1	35	39	0
162	25	22	6	2	44	48	0	186	57	33	6	0	24	28	0
163	25	22	1	2	45	48	0	187	21	15	0.5	1	39	43	0
164	14	79	3	1	45	47	0	188	57	33	1	0	25	29	0
165	14	79	2	1	47	51	0								
166	37	48	1	1	36	39	0								
167	49	64	0.75	1	46	50	0								
168	56	26	1	1	41	47	0								

10.6 Supplementary material

This chapter introduced a variety of transmission chain models to describe data on outbreaks in households of three susceptibles. In practice we are likely to need such models for households with a larger number of susceptibles. The following extends these models to households with four and five susceptibles.

10.6.1 Convenient notation for transmission chain models

We begin by introducing notation that avoids excessively complicated expressions for chain probabilities.

For Q, the probability that an individual avoids infectious contacts with a given infective from his household, we will write

$$\nu_{ij} \quad \text{for} \quad \mathrm{E}[Q^i(1-Q)^j].$$

It is important to remember that when Q varies, its variation has a different interpretation in the different models.

For notational convenience, arrows in the chain notation are omitted, so that the chain $1\to 2\to 1$ is simply written 121. This simpler notation is used in the three tables of transmission chain models given below.

10.6.2 Models for households with three susceptibles

To familiarize ourselves with this notation we summarize, in Table 10.15, the four different transmission chain models for households of size three that were introduced earlier in this chapter.

Table 10.15: *Chain model for a household of size 3 (1 initial infective)*

Chain	Chain binomial	Infectives differ	Susceptibles differ	Households differ
1	q^2	ν_{20}	ν_{10}^2	ν_{20}
11	$2\tilde{q}q^2$	$2\nu_{10}\nu_{11}$	$2\nu_{01}\nu_{20}$	$2\nu_{21}$
111	$2\tilde{q}^2q$	$2\nu_{01}\nu_{11}$	$2\nu_{01}\nu_{11}$	$2\nu_{12}$
12	$\tilde{q}^2$	ν_{02}	ν_{01}^2	ν_{02}

The model in column two of Table 10.15 assumes that there is no variation in Q and the common value is denoted q. We first met this model in Table 10.5. Its probabilities can also be expressed in terms of ν_{20}, ν_{21}, ν_{12} and ν_{02}, but we have not done so because expressions for its chain probabilities are not complicated. The model is referred to as chain-binomial because, as becomes clear below, each generation contributes a Binomial probability to the overall chain probability.

The model in column three of Table 10.15 assumes that an independent value is assigned to Q for each infective. For example, the duration of the infectious period may be different for infectives. Its chain probabilities are expressed in terms of ν_{10}, ν_{01}, ν_{20}, ν_{02} and ν_{11}. These are not five distinct parameters, since each of them can be expressed in terms of $q = \mathrm{E}(Q)$ and $\sigma^2 = \mathrm{Var}(Q^2)$, as in Table 10.7. The preference for using parameters q and σ^2, as in Table 10.7, lies in their interpretation as mean and variance. For larger households the ν_{ij} notation is more convenient.

Column four of Table 10.15 is the same model as that given in Table 10.9. It assumes that an independent value is assigned to Q for each susceptible, to reflect variation in the susceptibility of individuals.

Finally, the model in the last column of Table 10.15 allows Q to vary from household to household, but not within households. The model in Table 10.11 is the particular form of this model obtained when we assume that Q has a Beta distribution.

10.6.3 Models for households with four and five susceptibles

Corresponding chain transmission models for outbreaks in households of size four and five are given in Table 10.16 and Table 10.17, respectively.

Table 10.16: *Chain model for a household of size 4 (1 initial infective)*

Chain	Chain binomial	Infectives differ	Susceptibles differ	Households differ
1	q^3	ν_{30}	ν_{10}^3	ν_{30}
11	$3q^4\tilde{q}$	$3\nu_{20}\nu_{21}$	$3\nu_{01}\nu_{20}^2$	$3\nu_{41}$
111	$6q^4\tilde{q}^2$	$6\nu_{10}\nu_{11}\nu_{21}$	$6\nu_{01}\nu_{11}\nu_{30}$	$6\nu_{42}$
12	$3q\tilde{q}^2q_2$	$3\nu_{10}^2\nu_{12}$	$3\nu_{01}^2\nu_{30}$	$3\nu_{32}$
1111	$6q^3\tilde{q}^3$	$6\nu_{01}\nu_{11}\nu_{21}$	$6\nu_{01}\nu_{11}\nu_{21}$	$6\nu_{33}$
112	$3q^2\tilde{q}^3$	$3\nu_{02}\nu_{21}$	$3\nu_{01}\nu_{11}^2$	$3\nu_{23}$
121	$3q\tilde{q}^2\tilde{q}_2$	$3\nu_{12}(1-\nu_{10}^2)$	$3\nu_{01}^2(\nu_{10}-\nu_{30})$	$3(\nu_{12}-\nu_{32})$
13	$\tilde{q}^3$	ν_{03}	ν_{01}^3	ν_{03}

These extensions are fairly straightforward, but some explanations are helpful because a few assumptions are made. We begin with the model in column two of Table 10.16 and Table 10.17.

10.6.4 Chain-binomial model

Assume that individuals are homogeneous, as far as disease transmission is concerned, and that susceptibles make infectious contacts independently of each other.

For larger households it may happen that a susceptible is exposed to

Table 10.17: *Chain model for a household of size 5 (1 initial case)*

Chain	Chain binomial	Infectives differ	Susceptibles differ	Households differ
1	q^4	ν_{40}	ν_{10}^4	ν_{40}
11	$4q^6\tilde{q}$	$4\nu_{30}\nu_{31}$	$4\nu_{01}\nu_{20}^3$	$4\nu_{61}$
111	$12q^7\tilde{q}^2$	$12\nu_{20}\nu_{21}\nu_{31}$	$12\nu_{01}\nu_{11}\nu_{30}^2$	$12\nu_{72}$
12	$6q^2\tilde{q}^2q_2^2$	$6\nu_{20}^2\nu_{22}$	$6\nu_{01}^2\nu_{30}^2$	$6\nu_{62}$
1111	$24q^7\tilde{q}^3$	$24\nu_{10}\nu_{11}\nu_{21}\nu_{31}$	$24\nu_{01}\nu_{11}\nu_{21}\nu_{40}$	$24\nu_{73}$
112	$12q^4\tilde{q}^3q_2$	$12\nu_{12}\nu_{31}\nu_{10}^2$	$12\nu_{01}\nu_{11}^2\nu_{40}$	$12\nu_{63}$
121	$12q^3\tilde{q}^2q_2\tilde{q}_2$	$12\nu_{10}\nu_{22}(\nu_{10}^2-\nu_{20}^2)$	$12\nu_{01}^2\nu_{40}(\nu_{10}-\nu_{30})$	$12(\nu_{52}-\nu_{72})$
13	$4q\tilde{q}^3q_3$	$4\nu_{13}\nu_{30}$	$4\nu_{01}^3\nu_{40}$	$4\nu_{43}$
11111	$24q^6\tilde{q}^4$	$24\nu_{01}\nu_{11}\nu_{21}\nu_{31}$	$24\nu_{01}\nu_{11}\nu_{21}\nu_{31}$	$24\nu_{64}$
1112	$12q^5\tilde{q}^4$	$12\nu_{02}^2\nu_{21}\nu_{31}$	$12\nu_{01}\nu_{11}\nu_{21}^2$	$12\nu_{54}$
1121	$12q^4\tilde{q}^3\tilde{q}_2$	$12\nu_{12}\nu_{31}(1-\nu_{10}^2)$	$12\nu_{01}\nu_{11}^2(\nu_{20}-\nu_{40})$	$12(\nu_{43}-\nu_{63})$
113	$4q^3\tilde{q}^4$	$4\nu_{03}\nu_{31}$	$4\nu_{01}\nu_{11}^3$	$4\nu_{34}$
1211	$12q^2\tilde{q}^3q_2\tilde{q}_2$	$12\nu_{01}\nu_{22}(\nu_{10}^2-\nu_{20}^2)$	$12\nu_{01}^2\nu_{31}(\nu_{10}-\nu_{30})$	$12(\nu_{43}-\nu_{63})$
122	$6q^2\tilde{q}^2\tilde{q}_2^2$	$6\nu_{22}(1-2\nu_{10}^2+\nu_{20}^2)$	$6\nu_{01}^2(\nu_{10}-\nu_{30})^2$	$6(\nu_{22}-2\nu_{42}+\nu_{62})$
131	$4q\tilde{q}^3\tilde{q}_3$	$4\nu_{13}(1-\nu_{30})$	$4\nu_{01}^3(\nu_{10}-\nu_{40})$	$4(\nu_{13}-\nu_{43})$
14	$\tilde{q}^4$	ν_{04}	ν_{01}^4	ν_{04}

more than one infective of a given generation. There are two ways to accommodate this in the model. We can make an assumption about the way exposures to the infectives arise or we can add parameters to the model. For the moment we take the latter approach. Denote the probability that a given susceptible avoids infection when exposed to i infectives of a specific generation by q_i, $i = 1, 2, \ldots$. We assume that q_i does not vary from generation to generation, although this assumption can be relaxed. Let S_j be the number of susceptibles of the household exposed to the I_j infectives of generation j. For $j = 1, 2, \ldots$, these assumptions give

$$\Pr(I_{j+1} = x \,|\, S_j = s, I_j = i) = \frac{s!}{x!(s-x)!}\,(1-q_i)^x q_i^{s-x}, \qquad x = 0, 1, \ldots, s.$$

It follows that the probability of a given transmission chain is the product of probability terms from different Binomial distributions.

In order to apply this model in practice one needs to make two assumptions. Firstly, assume that there are no subclinical, or asymptomatic, infections, so that all cases can be recognized. Secondly, assume that after their infectious period infectives recover and acquire immunity for the remaining duration of the outbreak. That is, infectives play no further role in transmission once their infectious period ends. These assumptions allow us to deduce the number of individuals who remain susceptible at the end of each generation, by

$$S_{j+1} = S_j - I_{j+1}, \qquad j = 1, 2, 3, \ldots,$$

with the initial values $I_1 = i_1$ and $S_1 = s_1$ assumed known. This completes the model formulation.

To illustrate the computation of chain probabilities, suppose a household initially consists of four susceptibles and one introductory infective, so that $s_1 = 4$ and $i_1 = 1$. For this household, the above model formulation gives the probability of the transmission chain $1\to 1\to 2$ as

$$\begin{aligned}
\Pr(1\to 1\to 2) &= \Pr(I_2 = 1 \,|\, S_1 = 4, I_1 = 1)\Pr(I_3 = 2 \,|\, S_2 = 3, I_2 = 1) \\
&\quad \times \Pr(I_4 = 0 \,|\, S_3 = 1, I_3 = 2) \\
&= 4\,\tilde{q}_1\, q_1^3 \times 3\,\tilde{q}_1^2 q_1 \times q_2 \;=\; 12\,\tilde{q}_1^3 q_1^4 q_2.
\end{aligned}$$

In general the probability of transmission chain $i_1\to i_2\to\cdots\to i_r$ is given by

$$\Pr(i_1\to i_2\to\cdots\to i_r) = \frac{s_1!}{i_2!i_3!\cdots i_r!}\prod_{j=1}^{r}(1-q_{i_j})^{i_{j+1}} q_{i_j}^{s_{j+1}},$$

where $i_{r+1} = 0$ and consequently $s_{r+1} = s_r$.

This family of models has parameters q_i, $i = 1, 2, \ldots$, with the number of parameters for any outbreak depending on the initial number of susceptibles in the household. Chain probabilities for households of size three depend only on the parameter q_1. In column two of Tables 10.15, 10.16 and

10.17, we have written q for q_1 and $\tilde{q}$ for $\tilde{q}_1$, for notational convenience. The parameter q_2 enters expressions for chain transmission probabilities for households of size four. For households of size five the parameter q_3 enters as well.

The household outbreak size model corresponding to each of the chain transmission models given in Table 10.17 is easily derived. To obtain the probability for any given outbreak size one simply adds the probabilities of all chains with that outbreak size.

Two well-known models, each with just one parameter, are particular cases of the multi-parameter chain-binomial model.

Reed-Frost model

The first specific case of our model is the Reed-Frost model, for which

$$q_i = q^i \quad \text{for each } i.$$

It assumes that susceptibles make infectious contacts with an infective randomly and independently. For each susceptible the event of avoiding infection is independent, and the same, for each infective present. Under the Reed-Frost assumption all transmission chain probabilities are determined once we specify the value of the single parameter $q = q_1$. For this model, q is interpreted as the probability that a given susceptible avoids infection by a given infective over the entire duration of the infectious period of the latter.

Greenwood model

A second specific case of our model is the Greenwood model which makes the assumption

$$q_i = \begin{cases} 1 & \text{when } i = 0, \\ q & \text{for } i = 1, 2, \ldots. \end{cases}$$

The Greenwood model assumes that each susceptible household member avoids exposure to the pathogen independently and that pathogen is deposited around the household environment only when at least one infective is present. When one or more infectives are present, the amount of pathogen does not depend significantly on the number of infectives present at the time. This model also contains just one parameter. Its parameter q is interpreted as the probability that a given susceptible avoids infection by the infectives of a single generation, as long as the generation contains at least one infective.

10.6.5 Model with variable infectivity

In Section 10.3.1 we explained how to derive expressions for transmission chain probabilities when there is variation in the infectivity of infected individuals. The derivation is similar for larger households, but one new feature enters the calculations. An assumption is required about the nature of exposures when there is more than one infective in a generation. Here we make the Reed-Frost assumption, adapted to allow infectivity to vary among infectives. It is useful to clarify what this means by illustrating the derivation of a transmission chain probability with this feature.

Consider the transmission chain $1 \to 2 \to 1$ in a household of size five. For an infective X, let Q_X denote the probability that a given susceptible avoids infection by X. Label the primary infective A, the two first generation infectives B and C, and the second generation infective D. The conditional probability of the transmission chain $1 \to 2 \to 1$, given Q_A, Q_B, Q_C and Q_D, is

$$\Pr(1 \to 2 \to 1 \mid Q_A, Q_B, Q_C, Q_D) = 6Q_A^2(1-Q_A)^2 \times 2Q_BQ_C(1-Q_BQ_C) \times Q_D,$$

the product of three Binomial probabilities. The unconditional probability is obtained by taking expectations, treating Q_A, Q_B, Q_C and Q_D as independent random variables. This gives

$$\begin{aligned}\Pr(1 \to 2 \to 1) &= 12\,\mathrm{E}[Q_A^2(1-Q_A)^2] \\ &\quad \times [\mathrm{E}(Q_B)\mathrm{E}(Q_C) - \mathrm{E}(Q_B^2)\mathrm{E}(Q_C^2)]\,\mathrm{E}(Q_D) \\ &= 12\,\nu_{22} \times (\nu_{10}^2 - \nu_{20}^2) \times \nu_{10},\end{aligned}$$

which agrees with the expression given in Table 10.17.

The model for transmission chains in households of size three is presented in Table 10.7, in terms of the two parameters $q = \mathrm{E}(Q)$ and $\sigma^2 = \mathrm{Var}(Q)$. For households of size four the model requires three parameters. For example, $\mathrm{E}(Q)$, $\mathrm{E}(Q^2)$ and $\mathrm{E}(Q^3)$ could be used. To specify the model for a household of size five we need an additional parameter, for example $\mathrm{E}(Q^4)$. Chain frequency data for households of size four and five are not really rich enough to warrant more than two parameters. We suggest that a Beta distribution, given by a density function of the form

$$f(x) = \text{constant} \times x^{a-1}(1-x)^{b-1}, \qquad 0 < x < 1, \quad (a, b > 0),$$

be assumed for Q when data are available for households of size larger than three. The Beta distribution is convenient because use of

$$\nu_{ij} = \mathrm{E}\left[Q^i(1-Q)^j\right] = a^{(i)}b^{(j)}/(a+b)^{(i+j)}, \quad i, j = 1, 2, \ldots, \qquad (10.1)$$

where $a^{(i)} = a(a+1)\ldots(a+i-1)$, etc., leads to explicit expressions for the transmission chain probabilities in terms of a and b.

Substituting

$$a = q(\tilde{q}q\sigma^2 - 1) \qquad \text{and} \qquad b = \tilde{q}(\tilde{q}q\sigma^2 - 1)$$

gives chain probabilities in terms of the two parameters $q = \mathrm{E}(Q)$ and $\sigma^2 = \mathrm{Var}(Q)$ for any household size.

10.6.6 Model with variable susceptibility

Section 10.3.2 describes how to derive the chain probabilities for outbreaks in households of size three when susceptibility varies. Again, the corresponding derivation for larger households requires an assumption about the way infectious contacts occur when there is more than one infective in a generation. Here, too, we make the Reed-Frost assumption. The derivation is illustrated by finding the expression for the probability of the transmission chain 1→2→1 in a household of size five.

Infectivity is now the same for each infected person, but susceptibility differs among individuals. Let Q_X denote the probability that susceptible X avoids being infected by a given infective. There is one primary infective and we label the remaining four household members A, B, C and D. The conditional probability, given Q_A, Q_B, Q_C and Q_D, that "A and B are first-generation infectives, C is a second-generation infective and D avoids infection throughout," is

$$(1 - Q_A)(1 - Q_B)Q_C Q_D \times Q_D^2(1 - Q_C^2) \times Q_D.$$

The unconditional probability of this event is obtained by taking the expectation, treating Q_A, Q_B, Q_C and Q_D as independent random variables. This gives

$$\mathrm{E}(1 - Q_A)\,\mathrm{E}(1 - Q_B)\,\mathrm{E}(Q_C - Q_C^3)\,\mathrm{E}(Q_D^4) = \nu_{01} \times \nu_{01} \times (\nu_{10} - \nu_{30})\nu_{40}.$$

Finally, the probability of transmission chain 1→2→1 is given by

$$12\nu_{01}^2\nu_{40}(\nu_{10} - \nu_{30}),$$

as in Table 10.17, because there are twelve different ways that the four initial susceptibles can be selected to produce the chain 1→2→1.

In applications it is best to keep the number of parameters to two by assuming that Q, which varies over susceptibles, has the Beta distribution with moments ν_{ij} given by Equation (10.1). This too gives a model that can be expressed in terms of $q = \mathrm{E}(Q)$ and $\sigma^2 = \mathrm{Var}(Q)$ for every household size.

10.6.7 Variation among households

Now suppose that Q, the probability that the susceptible avoids being infected by the infective, is the same for each susceptible-infective pair of a given household. However, Q varies independently from household to household. Again we need to specify the way infectious contacts occur when there is more than one infective in a generation. Here, too, we make the Reed-Frost assumption.

Then the conditional probability of the chain 1→2→1 in a household of size five, given Q, is

$$\begin{aligned}
\Pr(1\!\to\!2\!\to\!1\,|\,Q) &= \Pr(I_2=2, I_3=1, I_4=0\,|\,Q, I_1=1) \\
&= \Pr(I_2=2\,|\,Q, I_1=1)\Pr(I_3=1\,|\,Q, I_2=2) \\
&\qquad \times \Pr(I_4=0\,|\,Q, I_3=1) \\
&= 6Q^2(1-Q)^2 \times 2Q^2(1-Q^2) \times Q \\
&= 12Q^5(1-Q)^2(1-Q^2).
\end{aligned}$$

Taking the expectation with respect to Q gives the unconditional probability

$$\Pr(1\!\to\!2\!\to\!1) = 12(\nu_{52} - \nu_{72}),$$

as in column five of Table 10.17.

To keep the number of parameters to two we assume that Q, which varies over households, has the Beta distribution with moments ν_{ij} given by (10.1), giving a model that can be expressed in terms of $q = \mathrm{E}(Q)$ and $\sigma^2 = \mathrm{Var}(Q)$.

10.7 Bibliographic notes

Norman Bailey stimulated greater interest in epidemic models and their use for analysis of infectious disease data with his 1957 book and its second edition, Bailey (1975). The material of this chapter builds on Bailey's analysis of transmission-chain data.

Terminology and notation

Terminology

Aggregated transmission intensity exerted by infective A
The transmission intensity A exerts on the group of current susceptibles

Aggregated transmission intensity a susceptible B is exposed to
The transmission intensity B is exposed to collectively from the group of current infectives

Basic reproduction number
Mean of the total number of individuals a typical infective infects when population immunity is negligible and no infectious disease control measures are in place

Branching process
Model describing the random dynamics of population growth when each individual produces offspring independently and growth is unbounded

Critical immunity coverage
Smallest fraction of community members that must be made immune to ensure an outbreak is minor (used with the assumption that all others are fully susceptible)

Critical vaccination coverage
Smallest fraction of community members that must be vaccinated to ensure an outbreak is minor

Cumulative transmission intensity function
A function describing the transmission intensity that has accumulated, over time, up to the current time

Delta Method
A method for computing the standard error of an estimate that is expressed in terms of another estimate with a known standard error

Effective reproduction number
Current value of the mean number of individuals a typical infective infects over his or her infectious period

Endemic transmission
Community transmission that is able to persist without repeated introduction of the infection

Epidemic
Outbreak in which the number of infectives builds up to a peak and then declines, leaving a substantial fraction of community members infected

Generation of infectives (or cases)
Group of infectives belonging to the same step in the transmission chain initiated by the primary infectives. Primary infectives make up Generation 1. The collection of their offspring is Generation 2.

Herd immunity
Immunity a susceptible acquires indirectly when a proportion of other community members is immunized

Homogeneous individuals
Individuals with the same susceptibility and infectivity characteristic

Household
Collection of individuals sharing an abode

Immunity coverage
Fraction of community members that is fully immune

Incubation period
Duration of time from infection until onset of symptoms in the host

Infectious agent
Microbial organism capable of causing disease, including bacteria, viruses, fungi and parasites

Infectious contact
Contact by an infective that is close enough for the infection to be transmitted if the contacted person has no immunity

Infectious period
Period of time during which the host sheds infectious agent and thereby is able to transmit the infection to others

Infective (noun)
Infected person, from the time of his infection until the end of his infectious period

Infectivity profile
A function capturing the *shape* of the infectivity of an infected individual over time since his infection, scaled so the area under its curve equals 1

Initial reproduction number
For a freshly introduced infectious disease, the mean number of individuals a primary infective infects over his, or her, entire infectious period

Latent period
Time period from the infection of a host until he sheds pathogen

Maximum likelihood estimate
Estimate of a parameter obtained by making the probability of the observed data as large as possible within the chosen class of models

Mean
Average of the values a random variable can take, with each value being weighted by its probability

Mode of a probability distribution
The value to which the largest probability is assigned

Offspring
Infected individuals generated by a specific infective

Offspring distribution
Probability distribution of the number of offspring generated by a specific infective

Outbreak
Collection of cases observed when an infection is newly introduced and subsequently fades out

Parameter
An unknown model constant that needs to be assigned a value by assumption or by estimation from data

Pathogen
Same as *infectious agent*

Primary or introductory infective
First infective of a fresh outbreak in a community

Primary household infective
First person infected in a given household

Random variable
Variable whose next realized value cannot be predicted with certainty

Reproduction number
See *basic*, *effective* or *initial* reproduction number

Secondary infective (or case)
Individual infected by a primary infective

Serial interval
Interval between the time of symptom onset in an infective and the time of symptom onset in his offspring

Susceptible (noun)
Individual susceptible to infection

Transmission chain
Enumeration of the generations of infectives, from Generation 1 (primary infectives) to the first generation to have zero offspring

Transmission intensity function
Quantification of the changing likelihood that infective A infects susceptible B over time since A was infected. See also aggregated and cumulative transmission intensity.

Transmission threshold property
A property of infectious disease transmission stating that epidemics can occur only when the value of a certain parameter is above 1.

Uniformly mixing
Each individual has the same chance to meet any other community member at all times

Vaccination coverage
Fraction of community members that is vaccinated

Notation

a	factor by which vaccination alters an individual's susceptibility
b	factor by which prior vaccination alters an infective's infectivity
$\mathrm{E}(X)$	expected value of random variable X
f_j	fraction of community members of Type j
H_j	number of households with j susceptible members
I_j	number of infectives in generation j
n	number individuals (or observations)
n_{S}	number susceptibles in the community
$N(t)$	number infected by time t
p_j	probability that an infective has j offspring
$\tilde{q}$	probability of infecting a given household partner, $\tilde{q} = 1 - q$
R	effective reproduction number (often at start of outbreak)
R_0	basic reproduction number
R_{H}	household reproduction number
R_{T}	reproduction number when there are types of individual
R^*	reproduction number following a public health intervention
$\mathrm{SD}(Y)$	standard deviation of the outbreak size
s.e.	standard error of an estimate
$S(t)$	number still susceptible at time t
t	calendar time; time since the start of an outbreak
u	time since the infective was infected
u_{L}	duration of the latent period
v	fraction of individuals vaccinated; vaccination coverage
$v^{\dagger}$	critical vaccination coverage
y	proportion of community eventually infected (deterministic)
Y	number of cases in an outbreak (stochastic)
μ	mean number of infectious contacts by one infective (outside his household)
ν	mean eventual size of an outbreak
ν_{H}	mean eventual size of the household outbreak resulting when a randomly selected susceptible is infected
ν_j	mean size of an outbreak initiated by one primary infective in a household that initially had j susceptibles
π	probability that an outbreak initiated by 1 infective is minor
σ	standard deviation of the offspring distribution
$\Psi(t)$	cumulative transmission intensity function
$\psi(u)$	transmission intensity between an infective-susceptible pair u time units after being infected
$\psi_{\Sigma}(u)$	aggregated transmission intensity function
$\omega(u)$	infective's infectivity profile u time units after his infection

References

Anderson, R.M. and May, R.M. (1991). *Infectious Diseases of Humans. Dynamics and Control.* Oxford University Press.

Athreya, K.B. and Ney, P.E. (2004). *Branching Processes.* New York: Dover.

Bailey, N.T.J. (1975). *The Mathematical Theory of Infectious Diseases and its Applications.* London: Griffin.

Ball, F.G. and Lyne, O.D. (2002). Optimal vaccination policies for stochastic epidemics among a population of households. *Mathematical Biosciences*, **177**, 333-354.

Ball F., Mollison, D. and Scalia-Tomba G. (1997). Epidemics with two levels of mixing. *The Annals of Applied Probability*, **7**, 46-89.

Bartlett, M.S. (1949). Some evolutionary stochastic processes. *Journal of the Royal Statistical Society, Series B*, **11**, 211-229.

Bartoszyński, R. (1972). On a certain model of an epidemic. *Applicationes Mathematicae*, **13**, 139-151.

Becker, N.G. (1977). On a general epidemic model. *Theoretical Population Biology.* **11**, 23-36. (correction: *ibid* **14**, 498.)

Becker, N.G. (1989). *Analysis of Infectious Disease Data.* CRC Press.

Becker, N.G. (1993). Martingale methods for the analysis of epidemic data. *Statistical Methods in Medical Research* **2**, 93-112.

Becker, N.G. and Dietz, K. (1995). The effect of household distribution on transmission and control of highly infectious diseases. *Mathematical Biosciences*, **127**, 207-219.

Becker, N.G. and Hall, R. (1996). Immunization levels for preventing epidemics in a community of households made up of individuals of various types. *Mathematical Biosciences*, **132**, 205-216.

Becker, N.G. and Starczak, D. (1997). Optimal vaccination strategies for a community of households. *Mathematical Biosciences*, **139**, 117-132.

Becker, N. G. and Starczak, D. (1998). The effect of random vaccine response on the vaccination coverage required to prevent epidemics. *Mathematical Biosciences*, **154**, 117-135.

Becker, N.G. and Utev, S. (1998). The effect of community structure on the immunity coverage required to prevent epidemics, *Mathematical Biosciences*, **147**, 23-39.

Britton, T. (1998). Estimation in multitype epidemics. *Journal of the Royal Statistical Society, Series B*, **60**, 663-679.

Britton, T. and Becker, N.G. (2000). Estimating the immunity coverage required to prevent epidemics in a community of households. *Biostatistics*, **1**, 389-402.

Caley, P., Philp, D.J. and McCracken, K. (2008). Quantifying social distancing arising from pandemic influenza. *Journal of The Royal Society Interface*, **5**, 631-639.

Cauchemez, S., Ferguson, N. M., Wachtel, C., Tegnell, A., Saour, G., Duncan, B. and Nicoll, A. (2009). Closure of schools during an influenza pandemic. *The Lancet Infectious Diseases*, **9**, 473-481.

Cauchemez, S., Valleron, A. J., Boelle, P. Y., Flahault, A. and Ferguson, N. M. (2008). Estimating the impact of school closure on influenza transmission from Sentinel data. *Nature*, **452**, 750-754.

Farrington, P. (2003). *Modelling Epidemics.* Open University Worldwide Ltd.

Ferguson, N.M., Cummings, D.A., Fraser, C., Cajka, J.C., Cooley, P.C. and Burke, D.S. (2006). Strategies for mitigating an influenza pandemic. *Nature*, **442**, 448-452.

Glass, K. and Barnes, B. (2007). How much would closing schools reduce transmission during an influenza pandemic? *Epidemiology*, **18**, 623-628.

Glass, R.J., Glass, L.M., Beyeler, W.E. and Min, H.J. (2006). Targeted social distancing design for pandemic influenza. *Emerging Infectious Diseases*, **12**, 1671-1681.

Hall, R. and Becker, N.G. (1996). Preventing epidemics in a community of households. *Epidemiology and Infection*, **117**, 443-455.

Halloran, M.E., Longini, I.R. and Struchner, C.J. (2010). *Design and Analysis of Vaccine Studies.* New York: Springer.

Halloran, M.E., Struchiner, C.J. and Longini, I.M. (1997). Study designs for evaluating different efficacy and effectiveness aspects of vaccines. *American Journal of Epidemiology*, **146**, 789-803.

Harris, T.E. (2002). *The Theory of Branching Processes.* Courier Dover Publications.

Heasman, M.A. and Reid, D.D. (1961). Theory and observation in family epidemics of the common cold. *British Journal of Preventive and Social Medicine*, **15**, 12-16.

Jewell, N.P. and Shiboski, S.C. (1990). Statistical analysis of HIV infectivity based on partner studies. *Biometrics*, **46**, 1133-1150.

Kendall, D.G. (1956). Deterministic and stochastic epidemics in closed populations. *Proceedings of the 3rd Berkeley Symposium on Mathematical Statistics and Probability*, **4**, 149-165.

Kermack, W.O. and McKendrick, A.G. (1927). A contribution to the mathematical theory of epidemics. *Proceedings of the Royal Society of London, Series A*, **115**, 700-721.

Ma, J. and Earn, D. J. (2006). Generality of the final size formula for an epidemic of a newly invading infectious disease. *Bulletin of Mathematical Biology*, **68**, 679-702.

Mott, J.L. (1963). The distribution of the time-to-emptiness of a discrete dam under steady demand. *Journal of the Royal Statistical Society B*, **25**, 137-139.

Rodrigues-da-Silva G., Rabello S.I. and Angulo, J.J. (1963). Epidemic of variola minor in a suburb of São Paulo. *Public Health Reports*, **78**, 165-171.

von Bahr, B. and Martin-Löf, A. (1980). Threshold limit theorems for some epidemic processes. *Advances in Applied Probability*, **12**, 319-349.

Wallinga, J. and Teunis, P. (2004). Different epidemic curves for severe acute respiratory syndrome reveal similar impacts of control measures. *American Journal of Epidemiology*, **160**, 509-516.

Waugh, W.A.O'N. (1958). Conditioned Markov processes. *Biometrika*, **45**, 241-249.

White, L.F. and Pagano, M. (2008). Transmissibility of the influenza virus in the 1918 pandemic. *PLoS ONE*, **3**, e1498.

Whittle, P. (1955). The outcome of a stochastic epidemic — a note on Bailey's paper. *Biometrika*, **42**, 116-122.

World Health Organization (1971a). Smallpox surveillance. *The Weekly Epidemiological Record*, **46**, 376-379.

World Health Organization (1971b). The smallpox situation. *WHO Chronicle*, **25**, 396-401.

Subject index

Age at infection, 161, 162, 164–165, 168, 183
Assumption,
  Greenwood, 182, 192
  Reed-Frost, 182, 192–194
  goodness-of-fit, 171, 173, 177–178, 180–182
Attack rate, 124–147
Basic reproduction number (R_0), 10, 39, 112, 124, 161
Beta distribution, 179, 189, 193–195
Binomial distribution, 31, 43, 69, 85, 170, 175, 188, 191, 193
Biology-based model, 83
Borel-Tanner distribution, 16, 24, 25, 35
Branching process, 5, 13, 30, 68, 197
Chain-binomial model, 181, 188, 189–192
  application to common cold, 182
  chain probabilities, 181–182, 188
  multi-parameter, 181
  parameter estimation, 182
  test of assumptions, 182
Chicken pox, 21
Common cold, 13, 182
Community of households, 37–54, 60–64, 66, 69, 73, 75, 77–79, 85–86, 95–99, 101–102
Critical vaccination coverage, 9, 43, 44, 58, 64
Crowding, 11, 179, 180, 182
Deterministic model, 25, 123, 124, 126, 139, 144, 146, 151, 162, 166
Distribution,
  Beta, 179, 189, 193–195
  Borel-Tanner, 16, 24, 25, 35
  Geometric, 17–18, 21, 29, 33–35, 127–128, 130
  Offspring,
    general, 8, 16, 17, 19, 45
  Poisson, 15–18, 21, 23–24, 27, 33, 88–89, 121, 140, 155–156
  Trinomial, 170, 172
  Weibull, 156–157
Ebola, 1
Effective reproduction number, 20, 106, 131, 161
Elimination of infection, 3, 46, 165
Endemic transmission, 22, 160, 164–166, 168
Epidemic,
  completely observed, 183
  curve, 151–167
  preventing, 5, 7–9, 28, 39, 40, 47, 63, 65, 91, 95, 105, 116, 124, 161
  probability of, 16, 24, 139
  size, 26, 121–125, 132, 139, 144–146
Epidemiological hypotheses,
  Greenwood, 182, 192
  heterogeneity
    in households, 179–180
    in infectivity, 91, 93–97, 176–177, 192–193
    in susceptibility, 58, 91–92, 97, 177–178, 194
  Reed-Frost, 182, 192–194
Generations of infectives, 12, 21, 34, 68, 153, 174
Geometric distribution, 17–18, 21, 29, 33–35, 127–128, 130
Goodness of fit, 171, 173, 177–178, 180–182
Greenwood assumption, 182, 192
Herd immunity, 125, 128–130, 135–137, 140
HIV, 1, 73

Homogeneous,
  individuals, 5, 61, 94, 108, 121, 123, 133, 172
  infectives, 7, 8, 40
Household,
  community of, 37–54, 60–64, 66, 69, 73, 75, 77–79, 85–86, 95–99, 101–102
  outbreak, 38, 46, 49, 50, 84, 96, 169–182
    mean size of, 39, 46, 50, 69
  transmission chain, 174–195
Immunity, 31, 95, 128, 135, 140
  coverage, 64, 95
    see also vaccination coverage
  community, 95
  herd, 125, 128–130, 135–137, 140
Incubation period, 198
  see also symptoms onset
Infection,
  potential, 7, 8, 37, 38, 110
  rate, *see* transmission rate
Infectious contact, 2, 12, 31, 70
  definition, 2
  not observed, 73, 96
Infectious period, 2, 10, 19, 72, 92, 108
  definition, 2, 72
Infective (noun), 2, 7, 38, 75, 93, 106, 112
  generations of, 12, 21, 34, 68, 153, 174
  primary
    community, 7, 19, 37, 45, 61, 69, 76, 97, 112, 156
    household, 39, 48, 61, 78, 111, 119
Infectivity, 72, 93–101, 134, 140
  profile, 78
  variation in, 176–177, 192
Latent period, 2, 20, 72, 76, 87, 92, 110, 152, 160
  definition, 20, 72
Martingale, 147, 149, 150
Mass immunization, 40, 57, 94, 125, 128, 136
Measles, 21, 22, 49, 73, 85–86, 169–180, 184
Minor outbreak, 13
  community of households, 37–54
  homogeneous infectives, 7–36
  types of individual, 55–60
    with households, 60
Model,
  adequacy, 169, 171, 173, 175, 177, 178, 180
  chain-binomial, 181, 188, 189–192
  goodness-of-fit, 171, 173, 177–178, 180–182
  parameter, 3, 6, 17, 35, 39, 46, 57, 62, 65, 74, 78, 105, 134, 138, 154, 158, 172
    estimation of, 20–23, 34–36, 46, 74, 75, 96, 130, 138, 147, 160–163, 168, 169–180
  variable, 3
Offspring, 8, 9
  distribution general, 8, 16, 17, 19, 45
  mean number, 8, 10, 32, 39, 55, 57, 58, 60, 68, 87
  modified allocation, 37
Outbreak size
  community, 14–15, 16, 22, 32, 44, 139
  household, 50, 97, 169–175
Parameter, 3, 6, 17, 35, 39, 46, 57, 62, 65, 74, 78, 105, 134, 138, 154, 158, 172
  estimation of, 20–23, 34–62, 46, 74, 75, 96, 130, 138, 147, 160–163, 168, 169–180
  threshold, 8, 25, 40, 56, 60, 68, 146
Poisson distribution, 15–18, 21, 23–24, 27, 33, 88–89, 121, 140, 155–156
Potential to infect, 7, 8, 37, 38, 110
Probability of avoiding infection, 75, 86, 91–94, 102, 147, 192–192
Public health intervention, 8, 40, 47, 57, 94, 103–115, 121, 125, 128, 136
Reed-Frost assumption, 182, 192–194
Reproduction number, 9
  basic, 10, 39, 112, 124, 161
  effective, 20, 106, 131, 161

- estimation of, 20–23, 34, 46, 130, 147, 159, 161
- household, 38, 40, 50, 60, 62, 69, 101, 111, 112, 118
  - basic, 39
- initial, 11, 87, 122, 130, 147, 159
- notation for, 12
- types of individual, 57, 59

SARS, 1, 3, 11, 107
Serial interval, 27, 73, 156–160
Size of outbreak,
- community, 14–15, 16, 22, 32, 44, 139
  - distribution, 16
- household, 50, 97, 169–175
  - distribution, 169–175

Smallpox, 3, 20–22, 157–160
Social distancing, 103–115
- ban on mass gathering, 103, 116, 143
- onset of symptoms, 21, 27, 73, 79, 103, 107–109, 112, 156, 183
- quarantining households, 103, 110, 111, 113, 118
- reduced mixing, 104–106

Stochastic model, 80, 122, 131, 139, 145, 147
Survey, 106, 118, 161
Susceptible (noun), 2, 86, 91, 177, 194
Symptoms
- onset, 21, 27, 73, 79, 103, 107–109, 112, 156, 183
- symptomatic period, 106, 108, 112, 156

Threshold
- parameter, 9
- property, 8, 25, 40, 56, 60, 68, 146

Transmission,
- chain, 174, 176–180, 182, 188–190
  - data, 175, 177, 178, 180, 182
  - definition, 174
- intensity, 3, 71, 71–88, 92, 94, 104, 107, 110, 132
  - aggregate exerted, 4, 76
  - aggregate exposed to, 4, 144
  - cumulative, 4, 76
  - function, 71, 71–80, 85, 110
- rate, 12, 25, 40, 71–89, 91
- threshold property,
  - uniformly mixing community, 8
  - community of households, 40
  - with types, 56, 60

Trinomial distribution, 170, 172
Uniform mixing, 5, 87, 88, 94, 108
Vaccination coverage, 9, 95, 134, 136, 147
- critical, 9, 43, 44, 58, 64

Vaccine effect, 92, 94, 101, 102
- on infectivity, 93, 96, 97, 102, 134, 136
- on susceptibility, 91, 96, 97, 102, 134, 136

Vaccine efficacy, 95
Weibull distribution, 156–157